D1357578

BRUNONIANISM IN BRITAIN AND EUROPE

(Medical History, Supplement No. 8)

BRUNONIANISM IN BRITAIN AND EUROPE

edited by

W. F. BYNUM and ROY PORTER

(*Medical History*, Supplement No. 8)

LONDON
WELLCOME INSTITUTE FOR THE HISTORY OF MEDICINE
1988

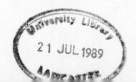

ISBN 0 85484 075 3
ISSN 0025 7273 8

Supplements to *Medical History* may be obtained at the Wellcome Institute for the History of Medicine, 183 Euston Road, London NW1 2BP; or by post from Professional and Scientific Publications, BMA House, Tavistock Square, London WC1H 9JR, U.K.

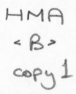

CONTENTS

ACKNOWLEDGEMENTS

This collection of papers arose out of a conference on the history of Brunonian medicine held at the Wellcome Institute for the History of Medicine, London, on 27 March 1987. The editors would like to express their thanks to those who contributed papers to that occasion and who have revised their essays for this volume, and to the Wellcome Trust for providing the funds which made that occasion possible.

INTRODUCTION

The English-speaking world finds it hard to reconcile that John Brown whose medical philosophy wins respectful mention in the Preface to Hegel's *Phenomenology* with the outlandish, opium-addicted Scottish medical teacher who died two hundred years ago. In part this difficulty arises because the events of Brown's own life, first as an obscure tutor, and then as a fringe medical teacher in Edinburgh, remain—and surely *will* remain—veiled in obscurity. His own papers have not survived, and most of what we do know of him is anecdotal—indeed (as Lawrence shows below) consists of highly contested anecdote.

Not least, wherever we look, we seem confronted with profound paradoxes. Brown set himself up in opposition to what historians acknowledge to have been the most powerful tradition of medical philosophy and practice hitherto generated in Britain, the Edinburgh school, led by his one-time mentor and benefactor, William Cullen. In contrast to that highly subtle, clinically-based disciplinary matrix, which made exemplary use of the newly-founded Edinburgh Infirmary, Brown—a man, it seems, with rather limited bedside experience—championed a programmatically simplifying system of the kind that would commonly be labelled "quackish". What appeal to the best-trained cadre of young doctors could a system possibly have, that denied the reality of specific diseases, gave not a fig for the prized Edinburgh nosologies, and exultingly discarded the complex and highly variegated standard therapeutics based upon the experience of centuries?

And yet Brunonianism clearly had a powerful appeal. In Britain, as Barfoot and Porter show below, it won the wholehearted support at least of a small number of vocal practitioners, and gained a sympathetic hearing amongst numerous luminaries, not least Erasmus Darwin and Thomas Beddoes. On the Continent—in particular in the German-speaking territories and Italy—its impact was great, its appeal broad, and its effects enduring. So why was Brunonianism not consigned to immediate oblivion as mere quackery? What enabled it to influence a whole generation as a species of alternative medical epistemology and practice? This is the question which provides the stimulus, and rationale, for the present collection of essays.

There are no simple answers, and—as the contributors are at pains to point out—there is no *single* answer. Each particular medical and cultural milieu offered specific incentives for a certain section of the medical profession to espouse. In Edinburgh, espousing Brunonianism was often the choice of young Turks whose medical radicalism might be matched by a socio-political radicalism. In Austria, as Kondratas stresses, Brunonianism could seem to offer a progressive and systematic rational approach to therapeutics; amongst German intellectuals, Tsouyopoulos points out, Brown's doctrines could be commandeered to play an active role in Romantic philosophical debates on the nature of life. In many cases this amounted, in Risse's apt metaphor, to new wine in old bottles—Brunonian doctrines and practices were, as often as not, acceptable facets of the great medical tradition dressed up in new names and offered as a radical alternative. For that reason, the problematical absence of profound ideological controversy over Brunonianism in many places, such as

England, may simply register the fact that it was easy quietly to absorb the acceptable aspects of Brown's teachings, and just as quietly discard the others.

Much work remains to be done. In particular, we do not as yet have even the beginnings of a prosopography of the Brunonian disciples or a chronology of its rise and fall (or successful absorption). It is hoped that this collection will stimulate further work on this important yet enigmatic figure.

Medical History, Supplement No. 8, 1988: 1–21.

CULLEN, BROWN AND THE POVERTY OF ESSENTIALISM

by

CHRISTOPHER LAWRENCE*

In 1795 the Bristol physician, Thomas Beddoes, introduced his edition of John Brown's *The elements of medicine* with the remark "It was not unusual for Brown's disciples to disagree, when they were called upon for a strict interpretation of his principal tenets."[1] Over a hundred years later, the London doctor Benjamin Ward Richardson made a similar observation: "Each of the different commentators of the Brunonian hypothesis has given an interpretation according to his own reading of it."[2] In spite of the difficulties which they had identified, both Beddoes and Richardson elucidated what they understood to be the essence of Brunonianism, the medical system identified with the eighteenth-century Scottish physician, John Brown. The discovery of a variety of meanings in Brown's writings, which both Beddoes and Richardson pointed to, is not a phenomenon confined to the system itself. Brown's various biographers have also come to varying conclusions about the meanings of his behaviour and utterances during his life.[3]

Two of the most important sources for the life of Brown are the accounts by Thomas Beddoes, and that by Brown's son, William Cullen Brown. Beddoes's life appeared in 1795, prefixed to his edition of Brown's *Elements.* Beddoes stated that his life of Brown, or Bruno as he was sometimes called, was based on obituary notices and "communications" with Mr Wait, "late respectable rector of Dumfries School". He admitted to shortcomings in his biography, because "very little of the information I had reason to expect, has reached me."[4] Beddoes edited the works of Bruno ("my hero" as he called him) in order, he said, to procure assistance for Brown's impoverished family. In addition, he hoped that the new edition with "observations on the character and writings of John Brown" would be a "consolation to [other] men of genius, pining under poverty and neglect".[5] Hardly, it might seem, the basis for a hostile account. However, William Cullen Brown, in his

* Christopher Lawrence, MB, ChB, MSc, PhD, Wellcome Institute for the History of Medicine, 183 Euston Road, London NW1 2BP.

[1] John Brown, *The elements of medicine. A new edition, revised and corrected with a biographical preface by Thomas Beddoes M.D.,* London, J. Johnson, 1795, vol. 1, p. cxxxvii.

[2] Benjamin Ward Richardson, *Disciples of Aesculapius,* London, Hutchinson & Co., 1900, vol. 1, p. 253.

[3] I shall not deal here with very recent interpretations of Brown's life and teaching. Instead, I shall attempt to contextualize the interpretations of the biographers for whom Brunonianism was a medical movement with which it was necessary to engage intellectually, because it either posed a threat or was seen as an important advance.

[4] Brown, op. cit., note 1 above, pp. xxxvi–xxxvii.

[5] Ibid., pp. viii, xxxv–xxxvi.

life of his father which appeared nine years later in 1804, accused Beddoes of using "scanty material" and of stigmatizing his father in the following manner:

> ... his want of medical erudition confidently affirmed; his composition, both in Latin and English, vilified; the extent of his practice questioned; he is arraigned of bigotry and pedantry in his youth, and of irreligion and arrogance in advanced life ... his person ... is likened to that of the clumsy buffoon in Cervantes ... [6].

John Brown was born either in 1735 or 36 in the parish of Buncle in the county of Berwick in Scotland.[7] He was, according to his son, a child prodigy and, by the age of five, had read the whole of the Old Testament.[8] Of Brown's childhood the ostensibly hostile Beddoes observed, "I conclude that he was endowed with that quickness of sympathy and that sensibility to the charms of nature, which characterize the infancy of genius."[9] After attending the local school Brown was apprenticed to a weaver. He soon left this employment, however, and went to the nearby grammar school because, as his son put it, to one so "highly cultivated; it may be readily conceived how truly disgusting the sordid life of one of the lowest mechanical businesses must have proved."[10] Brown's biographers credit him with a reputation for great physical and mental strength in his grammar school years. Beddoes stated that he "had vigour of body with vigour of mind, and exerted both".[11] At some point in his youth he renounced the faith of the strict religious sect to which his family belonged. Beddoes recorded this with some relief since, as he put it, "I see not what should have hindered a man endowed with so acute and comprehensive a genius from attaining equal pre-eminence in polemical divinity."[12]

By 1755 Brown's reputation as a scholar gained him the position of tutor in a laird's household. Scarcely had he entered this post, however, than he left. In Beddoes's opinion Brown "did not long continue to be an agreeable inmate [because it] is likely enough that he added the stiffness of pedantry to the sourness of bigotry."[13] His son, on the other hand, concluded that Brown had left because "he was not treated with the respect due to his situation."[14] From here Brown went to Edinburgh to study divinity. He soon gave this up too, however, and turned his attention to medicine. For this period of Brown's life a third biographical source, John Thomson's *Life of William Cullen,* offers yet another interpretation of Brown's career. Thomson's work, written in the 1820s, had a perspective quite different from that of Beddoes or Brown's son, as Thomson made plain:

---

[6] John Brown, *The works of Dr John Brown M.D. To which is prefixed a biographical account of the author,* by W. C. Brown, 3 vols., London, J. Johnson, 1804, vol. 1, pp. v–vii.
[7] Brown's early biographers (including his son) give conflicting accounts of the date and village (variously Lintlaws or Preston) of his birth. His most recent serious student is definite about 1736 and Preston, but cites no other sources than the first accounts. See Guenter B. Risse, 'The history of John Brown's medical system in Germany during the years 1790–1806', Ph.D diss., University of Chicago, 1971, p. 69.
[8] Brown, op. cit., note 6 above, p. xix.
[9] Brown, op. cit., note 1 above, p. xxxvii.
[10] Brown, op. cit., note 6 above, p. xxvi.
[11] Brown, op. cit., note 1 above, p. xli.
[12] Ibid., p. xliv.
[13] Ibid., p. xlv.
[14] Brown, op. cit., note 6 above, p. xli.

It is in the first place to be observed, that the two biographical accounts of Dr Brown given by Dr Beddoes and by William Cullen Brown, the son of Dr Brown, contain so many erroneous statements, so many representations quite at variance with facts, that they may, without injustice, be pronounced to be rather agreeable romances, and extraordinary pieces of fiction, than genuine narratives of matters of fact.[15]

In spite of their differences, all three authors agree that during his first four or five years studying medicine at Edinburgh, Brown was admitted free by the professors to their lectures, that he taught Latin, and that he became a grinder or extramural coach and composer of theses. In 1765 Brown opened a boarding house. At this time, according to his son,

The pleasures of the table and the unconstrained hilarity he enjoyed at the convivial meetings of . . . [his] . . . companions, were by nature sufficiently agreeable to one of his vivacity of disposition and strong passions.[16]

Beddoes saw matters rather differently and suggested that Brown "seems to have given in to the most dangerous of vices".[17] Also during these years, his son relates, Brown, in consequence of his menial position, had to render himself "agreeable to those on whom his livelihood depended".[18] One of these was the popular and well-connected professor of medicine, William Cullen. Brown's son represented Cullen as the exploiter of his father's talents. He wrote that "Dr Cullen, who was extremely deficient in classical erudition, conceived the idea of turning his pupil's intimate knowledge of Latin to his own permanent advantage."[19] Beddoes took a similar view. John Thomson, however, had a rather different perception of the relationship:

It is stated, more or less distinctly, both by Dr Beddoes and by Dr C. Brown, that Dr Cullen found Mr John Brown's knowledge of the Latin language useful, and made him a sort of amanuensis or Latin secretary. This is entirely a piece of invention. The only capacity in which Dr Cullen employed Mr John Brown was as tutor or private teacher to his children, to assist them in the preparation of their lessons and their Latin exercises.[20]

Thomson further professed incomprehension that Beddoes could possibly think that a man as great as Cullen would employ, as an amanuensis, a man who was little more than an adept at the art of "low buffoonery".[21]

The events following Brown's association with Cullen are the subject of striking differences of interpretation among the biographers. According to Brown's son and Beddoes, Cullen had promised to exert his interest on Bruno's behalf for the first

[15] John Thomson, *An account of the life, lectures and writings of William Cullen M.D.*, Edinburgh, William Blackwood and Sons, 1859, vol. 2, p. 710. This work was actually completed by Thomson's son William and by David Craigie, but for the purposes of the present paper the book can be considered a single-authored text, since these other two authors completed the book by using Thomson's manuscripts.

[16] Brown, op. cit., note 6 above, p. lii.

[17] Brown, op. cit., note 1 above, p. li.

[18] Brown, op. cit., note 6 above, p. liii.

[19] Ibid., p. lv.

[20] Thomson, op. cit., note 15 above, vol. 2, p. 711. Thomson defended Cullen's knowledge of Latin. Interestingly, it had been called into question before, at the time of Cullen's bid for the chair of the Practice of Physic. See [Anon], *A letter from a citizen of Edinburgh to Doctor Puff*, Edinburgh, 1764, p. 11.

[21] Thomson, op. cit., note 15 above, p. 713.

vacant University chair and, accordingly, in 1776 Brown put himself forward for the chair of the Institutes of Medicine.[22] Beddoes contended that Cullen, on being shown the name of Brown in the list of candidates, is said to have exclaimed in the "vulgar dialect" of the country *"Why sure this can never be our Jock!"*[23] Beddoes was here suggesting that the urbane Cullen was stigmatizing Brown as a rustic and thus wholly inappropriate to aspire to an Edinburgh Chair and the polite social world to which it gave entry. Thomson, however, denied the suggestion that Cullen had ever encouraged Brown and, indeed, claimed that the Town Council records showed that Brown had never been a candidate for the chair.[24] Following this episode there was at least one further serious disagreement between Cullen and Brown. Brown put his name forward for election to the prestigious Edinburgh Philosophical Society and was duly blackballed. According to Thomson, Cullen had advised Brown, for his own good, "to withdraw his application".[25] Brown's son, however, held that his father's rejection was negotiated by Cullen, jealous of his own originality and "dreading the shock, which his own favourite opinions . . . would sustain . . . from a rival".[26] The result, Beddoes stated, was that "Cullen estranged the mind of his Latin secretary" or, as Thomson observed, "Cullen ceased to hold any communication with him; it is said even to mention his name."[27] Following the breach between the two men, Brown began to teach his own system of medicine in Edinburgh in opposition to that of Cullen, and in 1780 he published the *Elementa medicinae* and, anonymously in 1787, *Observations on the principles of the old system of physic*. Another Brunonian work, *An inquiry into the state of medicine,* was published in 1781 under the name of Robert Jones, although Brown's son stated that the work was written by his father since it was a *"moral certainty"* that it could not have been the production of Jones.[28]

Brunonianism certainly caused a stir. Its adherents created havoc with the intellectual life of Edinburgh, especially in the 1780s in the students' Royal Medical Society and in the Royal Infirmary.[29] There can be no doubt either of the rancour which the controversy generated on both sides, nor the violence with which the dispute was pursued. Brown's son accused "Dr Cullen and his abettors" of being "ungenerous and disgraceful" and of attempting to "crush the doctrine, and involve its author and his family in ruin".[30] Beddoes, a trifle less sympathetic, noted "as the Cullenian hypotheses were sinking into disrepute, many of the ablest students resorted to the standard of Brown, . . . it was joined also by the most idle and dissolute."[31]

The remainder of Brown's life in Edinburgh was as colourful as his early career. In 1784 or 1785, he established a Masonic institution, 'The Lodge of the Roman Eagle', with the noble intention, said his son, of preventing the decline of Roman language and

---

[22] Brown, op. cit., note 6 above, p. lviii.

[23] Brown, op. cit., note 1 above, p. lvii.

[24] Thomson, op. cit., note 15 above, p. 712.

[25] Ibid., p. 715.

[26] Brown, op. cit., note 6 above, p. lxiv.

[27] Brown, op. cit., note 1 above, p. lix; Thomson op. cit., note 15 above, p. 715.

[28] Brown, op. cit., note 6 above, p. clxvii. Michael Barfoot argues convincingly that Jones was the author (personal communication); see also Michael Barfoot, this volume.

[29] For the local political meanings of the Brunonian controversy see Michael Barfoot, this volume.

[30] Brown, op. cit., note 6 above, p. lxxv.

[31] Brown, op. cit., note 1 above, p. lxii.

literature.[32] Beddoes less generously suggested that Brown saw that the medical students' interest in Freemasonry "afforded him a chance of proselytes".[33] In 1786, according to Thomson, Brown, in "straitened circumstances, and in debt" moved to London, where he died, after a spell of imprisonment, in 1788, aged about fifty-two.[34] Beddoes recorded that "he died, if I am not misinformed, in the night, having swallowed as he went to bed a very large dose of laudanum; a species of dram to which he had indeed been long addicted."[35]

All these authors, including the hostile Thomson, developed the view that Brown's character, or perhaps rightly, his charisma, was the foundation of the attraction of his teachings, both to students and others. They also concur in the opinion that this charisma was fuelled by the consumption of large amounts of brandy and opium. The charisma, however, was not universally effective. Beddoes recorded that, after encountering Brown in 1782 "I never desired his conversation a second time." He spoke, said Beddoes, with a "Doric dialect" which "had nothing prepossessing to an English ear. It was so broad as to leave me often uncertain of what he said."[36] Beddoes also gave an equally unsympathetic account of a Brunonian evening:

> One of his pupils informs me that when he found himself languid, he sometimes placed a bottle of whisky in one hand, and a phial of laudanum on the other; and that, before he began his lecture, he would take forty or fifty drops of laudanum in a glass of whisky; repeating the dose four or five times during the lecture. Between the effects of these stimulants and voluntary exertion, he soon waxed warm, and by degrees his imagination was exalted into phrenzy.[37]

His son, however, denied the charges of gross indulgence and claimed that his father's "intemperate excesses" were "egregiously exaggerated", and that "many ridiculous stories of the frolics committed by him in a state of ebriety have been circulated at his expense."[38] But Bruno, as even his son admitted, "was rather free in his religious sentiments" and also had unconventional political allegiances.[39] Beddoes recorded that "Brown was the first person I ever saw absurd enough to profess himself a Jacobite."[40] His son, however, rendered this undeniable association honourable by claiming that no one should be surprised that "a cause which has induced the most honourable and bravest chieftains in Scotland disinterestedly to draw their swords should have been espoused by a man of his warmth."[41]

Although they agreed on many details, these earliest biographers of Brown differed considerably in their interpretations of his actions. This is hardly surprising since they wrote from quite different social and personal perspectives. In the instance of Brown's son, the defence of his father's behaviour would seem to lie in the filial relationship. In the case of Thomson and Beddoes, their differing accounts seem to be

---

[32] Brown, op. cit., note 6 above, p. lxxix.
[33] Brown, op. cit., note 1 above, p. lxxxv.
[34] Thomson, op. cit., note 15 above, p. 716.
[35] Brown, op. cit., note 1 above, p. xciii.
[36] Ibid., p. lxxx.
[37] Ibid., p. lxxxvii.
[38] Brown, op. cit., note 6 above, p. cxxxiii.
[39] Ibid., p. cxxxviii.
[40] Brown, op. cit., note 1 above, p. lxxxi. For the local meanings of this association see Barfoot, this volume.
[41] Brown, op. cit., note 6 above, p. cxli.

related to their diametrically opposed political positions. However, not only were their accounts of Brown's life at variance, so were their interpretations of his system as well as that of Cullen. These differences also derived from their political philosophies. Before Beddoes and Thomson engaged with Brunonianism, however, there had been other accounts of the system.

In an account published one year after the *Elementa medicinae* of 1780, Brown himself, or more likely his close friend Robert Jones, described the core or crucial achievement of the system. This Jones represented as the first, correct application of the method of natural philosophy to medicine. A fundamental feature of this method was described by the Newtonian axiom that causes should not be multiplied and, Jones noted, "The application of this invaluable precept to medicine was discovered by Dr Brown."[42] By properly applying the method of induction Brown had been able to reduce "the whole phaenomena of life . . . to one simple cause . . . excitability".[43] This he did by first observing the simplest of medical phenomena, health itself, and then ascending to examine disease, which exhibits "the most complex phaenomena, as referable to man". However, unlike other inquirers, at no point did Brown invoke new causes for these more complicated states. "This", said Jones of the system, was "a view of the animal-oeconomy equally new and scientific".[44] In this text, therefore, Jones represented the essential feature of Brunonianism as being the recognition that the causes of health were the same as the causes of disease. Jones considered that Brown had achieved a feat comparable with that of Newton. He had arrived at "the most universal conception the mind can attain . . . *That is that all powers operating upon the animal and vegetable kingdoms, and creative of all their phaenomena, stimulate.*"[45] From this, quite properly, followed the deduction that specific therapies were absurd. For since stimulation is the only power that can act on the body, what is actually curing the patient when a physician prescribes a so-called specific is simply stimulation, not some specific property of the drug. Thus Brown had recognized that the use of specifics was actually a variety of that most heinous of medical practices, empiricism. Giving a specific drug implied a specific disease, and to account for specific diseases physicians employed a "multiplicity of causes". Whereas in Brown's system "The cause he assigns is one . . . a variation in the degree of excitement."[46] Brown's philosophy, Jones continued, necessarily demonstrated that nosology was a false science, because it was based on the fundamental methodological error that diseases with similar symptoms have similar causes and diseases with dissimilar symptoms, dissimilar causes. Whereas, of course, there was only one cause of disease, a change in excitability.

The *Inquiry* was thus a text which represented the crucial or essential nature of Brunonianism to be its systematic character, resting on the correct application of a

[42] Robert Jones, *An inquiry into the state of medicine on the principles of inductive philosophy*, Edinburgh, T. Longman and T. Cadell, London, C. Elliott, 1781, p. 86. For more details of Jones's life see Michael Barfoot, this volume. On its authorship see note 28 above: for present purposes authorship is unimportant, since both Brown and Jones were committed to challenging Edinburgh medicine on its own ground.

[43] Jones, op. cit., note 42 above, p. 93.

[44] Ibid., pp. 37–8.

[45] Ibid., p. 71.

[46] Ibid., pp. 85–7. Brown is attacking here the categories of predisposing, accessory, and proximate causes.

number of philosophical principles attributed to Newton. Effectively all the details of the system are deducible from these principles. Now systematic medicine was the basis of professional teaching in Edinburgh and knowledge of a system based on philosophical principles, identified with Newton, was taught by all the professors to be the hallmark of the rational or dogmatic physician.[47] In keeping with this, the professors also taught that empiricism was the most contemptible of medical philosophies. Brown was educated within this tradition and, amongst other things, his attempts to obtain an Edinburgh MD suggest that he identified with it.[48] It is also known, from both friendly and hostile sources, that Brown devised his *system* of medicine in opposition to that of Cullen, and that Brown taught his new *system* to the students. In this text, therefore, however apparently antagonistic to orthodox medicine it might seem, Jones, also medically educated in Edinburgh, was representing his friend's approach to medicine as falling squarely within the orthodox Scottish tradition. Indeed Jones argued, rather cleverly, that Brown's philosophy showed that previous Scottish systems were upholding the very philosophy they were designed to resist: empiricism. Thus Jones represented Brown in exactly the way that Cullen represented himself, as a supporter of the view that progress in medicine was to be achieved by employing fundamental philosophical principles in order to arrive at a general explanation graced by causal simplicity. Causal simplicity, in one way or another, was stipulated by such Scottish literati as David Hume, Adam Smith, and James Hutton as the cornerstone of a comprehensive and satisfying scientific explanation.[49] Thus Jones presented Brown's achievement as having *properly* practised medical theorizing as advocated by the great Scottish thinkers. In this text, Jones represented Brown not as a destroyer of the old medicine, but as a reformer who shared ground rules with Cullen and others about what medicine was and how it was to be improved. Indeed, he was representing Brown in much the same way that Cullen had portrayed his own relation to Boerhaave. The *Inquiry* was published in 1781, when Brown was still in Scotland and attempting to attract orthodox students away from the University and particularly from Cullen. Its representation of Brunonianism as a methodically-achieved dogmatic system based on Newtonian principles was, therefore, a locally-tuned intervention into the traditions of Edinburgh medicine.

Not everyone, however, saw its systematic nature to be the essential feature of Brunonianism. Indeed, one of the earliest published responses to Brown's work ignored altogether these pretensions to a systemic character. This attack was the anonymous *Observations on the medical practice of Dr. Brown,* which appeared in 1788. It was almost certainly written by a regular, English, provincial practitioner.[50] For this

[47] See Christopher Lawrence, 'Medicine as culture: Edinburgh and the Scottish Enlightenment', Ph.D. diss., University of London, 1984 and *idem,* 'Ornate physicians and learned artisans' in W.F. Bynum and Roy Porter (editors), *William Hunter and the medical world of the eighteenth century,* Cambridge University Press, 1985, pp. 153–76.

[48] He eventually received his degree from St. Andrew's.

[49] See Lawrence, op. cit., note 47 above. Also on Smith and Hume see J. R. R. Christie, 'The rise and fall of Scottish science' in Maurice Crosland (editor), *The emergence of science in Western Europe,* London, Macmillan Press, 1975, pp. 111–26. On Hutton see Roy Porter, *The making of geology,* Cambridge University Press, 1977.

[50] [John Leedes Hemingston], *Observations on the medical practice of Dr. Brown,* Ipswich, 1788. Hemingston is identified as the author in the British Library Catalogue. I have been unable to find any

author, the crucial part of the Brunonian doctrine was not its use of philosophical principles, but what he perceived as its radical therapeutic recommendations: in particular, that stimulants should be employed in inflammatory fevers. The author of the *Observations* was, medically speaking, a self-confessed conservative. He valued tradition and orthodoxy on the grounds that they necessarily embodied hundreds of years of accumulated experience. Further, orthodox wisdom was not primarily embodied in institutions or in books but in what physicians actually did at the bedside. Anything other than the most limited therapeutic innovation was, therefore, bad medicine. Eclecticism, gradual change, and deference to authority were themselves the signs that medicine was on its slow but sure path to "further improvement".[51] Thus for him the essence of Brown's work was its injunction to break with traditional *practice*. It was this which identified Brunonianism as a doctrine of a "singular and extraordinary nature". The most "conspicuous" part of this heresy was the recommendation that large doses of laudanum should be employed in fevers. This was a doctrine, the author remarked, which "surely, cannot but strike almost every person as uncommon and immoderate".[52] From this author's position, Brown's teaching represented "Credulity, fashion, the love of novelty, and a propensity to rush from one extreme to another".[53] Not surprisingly the author underwrote tradition by invoking authority, referring to the "learned and ingenious . . . Dr. Percival"; "that part of Dr. Cullen's works where he has so very ingeniously and satisfactorily discussed this subject"; "that truly ingenious man, Mr. John Hunter"; "those diligent observers of nature, Hippocrates and Sydenham"; "the elegant Celsus"; the "illustrious names, Cullen, Duncan and Gregory"; "that very learned and sagacious . . . Dr. George Fordyce", the "celebrated Sir John Pringle"; "the eminent Hoffmann" and, finally, "that celebrated professor, bright ornament of the medical profession, Dr. Cullen".[54] All of these great figures, he noted, avoided stimulants in inflammatory fevers, therefore, he deduced, this must be proper practice. Such prescribing, he said, "observe[d] due bounds" and "avoid[ed] those extravagant sallies which are generally looked upon to be the principal and leading marks of all extremes".[55]

The author thus identified himself with orthodoxy, and defined orthodoxy itself as traditional, unspectacular practice and cautious innovation. He argued that it was therapeutic innovation or, worse, therapeutic radicalism which brought the profession into disrepute. In the years around the turn of the century such activity was increasingly seen by regulars as the distinguishing sign of a populist, a flagrant self-advertiser, or even a quack. The *Observations,* therefore, did not represent Brown as an inside reformer, as the *Inquiry* had done, but as a dangerous outsider, a subverter of long-standing tradition. Such a response to Brunonianism might be expected from a provincial, English, surgeon-apothecary. At this time general practitioners were slowly

---

trace of this man. However, a Mr Leedes, a surgeon who practised in Hemingstone, Suffolk *c*.1790–1830, seems the most likely author: I am grateful to Dr D. van Zwanenberg for this information.

[51] Ibid., p. 5.

[52] Ibid., p. 7.

[53] Ibid., p. 20. Hemingston was quoting from Thomas Percival, *Essays medical and experimental,* 2nd ed., London, J. Johnson, 1757, p. 352.

[54] Hemingston, op. cit., note 50 above, pp. 7, 11, 14, 18, 21, 22, 29, 34.

[55] Ibid., p. 39.

creating their self-identity in the face of intense competition. To do this they used their shared education and their common practice as signs of their orthodoxy. Brunonianism, to this author, therefore represented the worst of possible threats, a regularly-trained doctor whose therapeutics seemingly made him indistinguishable from quacks.[56]

Other authors also saw striking innovation as the kernel of Brown's teaching. But some, for instance Thomas Beddoes, represented Brown's break with tradition as a virtue. Beddoes was a political radical and, in 1795, a year in which he was involved in anti-government agitation, he published a defence of Bruno's works which represented them as revolutionary texts.[57] Beddoes held that Brown's achievement was to have cut through the problem of the nature of life. Beddoes began, "Brown, avoiding all useless disquisition concerning the cause of *vitality,* confines himself to the phaenomena."[58] This was a significant reading. The similarity of Beddoes's description of Brown's work to the so-called materialistic doctrines of such French ideologues as Cabanis, with which Beddoes was very familar, is obvious.[59] In France the analysis of the *phenomena* of life was central to the ideologues' establishment of physiology as the fundamental science of mind and society. To the ideologues, speculation on unknown and unknowable causes of life was pointless (Beddoes's "useless disquisition"). A further feature of ideology was its use of environmentalism as the intellectual foundation of a system of medical police. Not surprisingly Beddoes, social reformer and educationalist, argued that until Brown "No writer had insisted so much upon the dependence of life on external causes."[60]

In his account of Brunonianism, Beddoes also addressed the suggestion that Brown's teaching had its origin in what Beddoes called the "obscure opinions of Dr Cullen".[61] Beddoes, however, had no confidence in this view. He quoted a sentence from Cullen which, so he said, had been used by others to prove Brown's plagiarism.

[56] On the appearance of the general practitioner and the importance of competitive threat, see Irvine Loudon, *Medical care and the general practitioner 1750–1850,* Oxford, Clarendon Press, 1986. For a suggestive model of the importance of therapeutics as the basis of identification among practitioners see John Harley Warner, *The therapeutic perspective. Knowledge and identity in America 1820–1885,* Cambridge MA, Harvard University Press, 1986. For a specific study of a therapeutic controversy between orthodox and irregular practitioners see Roy Porter, ' "I Think Ye Both Quacks": the controversy between Dr Theodor Myersbach and Dr John Coakley Lettsom', in W. F. Bynum and Roy Porter (editors), *Medical fringe and medical orthodoxy,* London, Croom Helm, 1987, pp. 56–78.

[57] On Beddoes's radicalism see Dorothy Stansfield, *Thomas Beddoes M.D. 1760–1808: chemist, physician, democrat,* Dordrecht, D. Reidel, 1984, especially chapters 6 and 7.

[58] Brown, op. cit., note 1 above, p. cxxxvi.

[59] On the ideologues see Erwin Ackerknecht, *Medicine at the Paris Hospital 1794–1848,* Baltimore, The Johns Hopkins Press, 1967; George Rosen, 'The philosophy of ideology and the emergence of modern medicine in France', *Bull. Hist. Med.,* 1946, **20:** 328–39. On Cabanis see Martin Staum, *Cabanis: Enlightenment and medical philosophy in the French Revolution,* Princeton University Press, 1980.

[60] Brown, op. cit., note 1 above, p. clix. On Beddoes on education and medical policing see Stansfield, op. cit., note 57 above, pp. 197–215. On medical police in France see L. J. Jordanova, 'Policing public health in France 1780–1815', in Teizo Ogawa (editor), *Public health,* Tokyo, Saikon, 1981, pp. 12–21. The use of Brunonianism by the various members of Beddoes's Bristol circle, in particular the young Humphry Davy, who was later an explicit vitalist, would make an interesting study: see Michael Neve, 'The young Humphry Davy: or John Tonkin's lament', in Sophie Forgan (editor), *Science and the sons of genius. Studies on Humphry Davy,* London, Science Reviews, 1980, pp. 1–32.

[61] Brown, op. cit., note 1 above, p. cxlvii.

Cullen had written, "It is probable that the nervous fluid in the brain, is truly capable of different states of excitement and collapse." To this, however, Beddoes added:

> In his youth, this author had imagined a mechanical hypothesis respecting the nervous fluid, which he regarded with fondness through life, and unfolded with great prolixity in the decline of his powers. When he wrote the passage I have quoted, his thoughts were turned from the living body to an electrical machine; and he evidently does no more than describe the common experiment, in which a congeries of flexible fibres is made to stand erect, and to diverge by electricity, and then shrinks together on the application of a conducting substance. His idea of excitement has therefore nothing in common with that of Brown.[62]

On Beddoes's reading, Cullen was an old-fashioned Boerhaaveian mechanist. This was a position which Beddoes reinforced by the argument that, before Brown, "investigations relative to medicine, had been carried on just as rationally as if to discover the qualities of the horse, the naturalist were to direct his attention to the movements of a windmill."[63] Beddoes's distinction between the ideas of Cullen and those of Brown was part of Beddoes's radical reading of Brown's text. Cullen was being associated with the past, the establishment, orthodoxy and tradition, and Brown was being identified, not with reform, as in the *Inquiry*, but with revolution.

Other radical readings of Brown's texts would make an interesting study. In particular, it might be rewarding to examine the ways in which authors interpreted Brown's view on the nature and seats of life. In the works of Cullen and other Edinburgh professors, the nervous system was designated as the fundamental source of *all* bodily sensation and motion, and the system through which *all* activity was mediated. Muscles were not designated as possessing autonomous irritability, as in Haller's system; rather, any apparent autonomous movement they showed was caused by residual nervous power. This model, I have suggested, was the medical view which corresponded to the Lowland literati's account of themselves as the élite managers of Scottish life.[64] Where Brown situated vitality was variously interpreted. In the *Inquiry*, Jones asserted that Brown's system "applies not only to animal but to vegetable life".[65] Democrats certainly interpreted Brown as having distributed vital power either throughout the body or at least as existing equally in the muscles and the nerves.[65] Beddoes proclaimed that Brown taught "Excitability is seated in the medullary portion of the nerves, and in the muscles".[66] Robert John Thornton, a Cambridge MD who had studied in Edinburgh, was probably another radical. By 1793 he was communicating the results of pneumatic experiments to Beddoes.[67] In a work published in 1795, he interpreted Brown in much the same way as Beddoes had done. He was more generous about Cullen than Beddoes had been, but Brown he regarded as

[62] Ibid., p. cxlvi.

[63] Ibid., p. clxi.

[64] Christopher Lawrence, 'The nervous system and society in the Scottish Enlightenment', in Barry Barnes and Steven Shapin (editors), *Natural order: historical studies of scientific culture*, Beverly Hills CA, Sage, 1979, pp. 19–40.

[65] Jones, op. cit., note 42 above, p. 87.

[66] Brown, op. cit., note 1 above, p. cxxviii.

[67] See Thomas Beddoes, *Letters from Dr Withering of Birmingham, Dr Ewart of Bath, Dr Thornton of London and Dr Biggs, late of the Isle of Santa-Cruz*, Bristol, Printed by Bulgin and Rosser, [n.d.]. Thornton's letter is dated 7 December 1793. See also William Munk, *The roll of the Royal College of Physicians of London*, 2nd ed., London, The College, 1828, vol. 3, p. 98.

"the father of the true science of medicine".[68] In particular, he praised Beddoes for his recognition that Brown was the first to deal with the phenomena of life, eschewing "unmeaning and vague terms".[69] Thornton wrote that Brown "attributed all the phenomena of life to the fibrous system, extending his doctrine to plants."[70] Similarly, Erasmus Darwin, who described Brown's *Elementa* as "a work of great genius" wrote of "the spirit of animation residing in the contracting fibres".[71]

Other authors also regarded Brown's text as revolutionary. They did not, however, see it as original. In the years of the French Wars, Thomas Morrison, Member of the Royal College of Surgeons of England, produced his *Examination into the principles of what is commonly called the Brunonian system*.[72] Morrison's text addressed both the Brunonian system, and the use which had been made of it by the physician and popular lecturer Thomas Garnett.[73] There can be little doubt about the community from which Morrison drew his perceptions of Brunonianism. "Brown", he began, "in his general acceptation [*sic*] of the word excitability appears evidently to mean the vital and mental principle of life and mind ... [and] ... I shall therefore wish the words Excitability, Vital Principle or Life to be considered synonimous [*sic*]."[74] But, he argued, Brown's description of the nature of the vital force was "confused, indistinct, and obscure".[75] Far from being a Newton of the living world, Brown had fundamentally misunderstood what a Newtonian explanation should look like. Life, the vital principle, said Morrison, was like gravity, ever constant and unchanging and the *cause* of vital actions. Brown, however, had designated life not only as a principle, but as the varying *effect* of stimuli on that principle. He had mistakenly identified the vital actions produced *by* the living principle with life itself. The cause of this error, said Morrison, lay in Brown's failure to recognize the importance of organization in living things. According to Morrison, Brown taught that stimuli acted directly on the vital principle and their action had no dependence on organization. But, said Morrison, "the very reverse of all this is the case; for it is only through the organization of the body that life exerts its powers."[76] Not surprisingly then, Morrison added, because

---

[68] 'A Friend to Improvements' [Robert John Thornton], *The philosophy of medicine*, 4th ed., London, C. Whittingham, 1799, vol. 1, p. 128.

[69] Ibid., p. 255.

[70] Ibid., p. 122.

[71] Erasmus Darwin, *Zoonomia; or the laws of organic life*, London, J. Johnson, 1794, vol. 1, pp. 74–5. Darwin's account of the relationship of the nerves to muscular motion is not easy to explicate and seems open to a number of readings; see ibid., pp. 7–11. Darwin certainly taught that plants had vital properties. For a very particular reading of Darwin see Maureen McNeil, *Under the banner of science: Erasmus Darwin and his age*, Manchester University Press, 1987, pp. 148–67.

[72] Thomas Morrison, *An examination into the principles of what is commonly called the Brunonian System*, London, Highley, [1806]. I have been unable to discover for certain who Morrison was. The title page designates him as "MRCS". There was a Surgeon-Apothecary Thomas Morrison who retired from the army in 1783: A. Peterkin and William Johnston, *Commissioned Officers in the medical services of the British Army 1660–1898*, London, The Wellcome Historical Medicine Library, 1968, entry 842.

[73] See T. Garnett MD, *A lecture on the preservation of health*, Liverpool, printed by J. M'creery, 1797. Garnett, a radical, had used the concept of excitability to present a view of life similar to that described by Beddoes. Since he did not actually produce an interpretation of the Brunonian system I have not dealt with him here. On this intriguing figure and for a bibliography see S. G. E. Lythe, *Thomas Garnett (1766–1802), Highland tourist, scientist and medical professor*, Glasgow, Polpress, 1984.

[74] Morrison, op. cit., note 72 above, pp. 14–15.

[75] Ibid., p. 26.

[76] Ibid., p. 42.

Brown was not interested in organization, "To the Brunonian System the knowledge of anatomy can be of no use . . . ".[77] Indeed, he scoffed, Brunonians will soon assert "the labours of anatomists are of very trifling moment."[78] Further, Brown, by his neglect of organization and his failure to understand the nature of the living principle, had fallen into the error of materialism, or, as Morrison put it: "His apprehension of being suspected of having material notions of life, seems to have proceeded from his really having such."[79]

There were, Morrison added, further difficulties with the system: "The laws of the animal economy are uniform and equal in all their effects, what is the strength of one power can never be the weakness of another."[80] Thus, he noted, the Brunonians foolishly explained the painful reaction of the eye kept in darkness and then exposed to the stimulus of bright light by postulating an accumulation of excitability.[81] But, Morrison argued, Brown had described an impossible situation: a small stimulus producing a great effect. The real reason for the response lay in the protective action of the eye muscles. Because of the *design* of the body, danger to the eye, indicated by pain, evokes the appropriate response. In his catalogue of Brown's errors, Morrison held that he had variously seated excitability, or the vital principle, in the nervous substance and muscles, or throughout the body's fibres. In either case the radical possibilities seemed clear to Morrison, who noted that Brown's view overlooked "The circulatory system . . . [which] . . . will be found to be perhaps more necessary to the action of excitability than the nervous."[82]

In the light of Morrison's explication of Brunonianism it is possible to offer a conjecture about the origin of his views. He was probably a London surgeon, and almost certainly a direct or distant disciple of John Hunter. Within the Hunterian school, the starting points of anatomical and physiological investigation were the existence of an autonomous and unknowable vital principle, the centrality of organization, and the importance of the blood and the vascular network. The methods of investigation were anatomical dissection and experiment; and the aims were, as Morrison put it, to trace "effects discernible in nature . . . to their great First Cause".[83] For Morrison, therefore, Brunonianism represented the very antithesis of all these things: it negated the importance of anatomy, it was materialist, irreligious, and thus potentially productive of the very worst social consequences. As he put it,

> The general conclusions of the Brunonian system lead to the most gross and false ideas of the nature of life and mind. The magnitude of this last objection, both in a physical and a moral point of view, is deserving of particular attention. The deplorable consequences which have arisen to society from the propagation of opinions connected with such erroneous notions, more especially in a neighbouring country, is too fresh in the minds of everyone to require repetition.[84]

[77] Ibid., p. 96.
[78] Ibid., p. 104.
[79] Ibid., p. 35.
[80] Ibid., p. 72.
[81] The example is used by Garnett, op. cit., note 73 above, p. 14.
[82] Morrison, op. cit., note 72 above, p. 21.
[83] Ibid., p. 131.
[84] Ibid., p. 126. On the revolutionary meanings of physiological texts in this period see Owsei Temkin, 'Basic science, medicine and the Romantic era', *Bull. Hist. Med.*, 1963, **37**: 97–129.

To a devout, presumably Tory, London surgeon, there was nothing new in Brunonianism. Here was something familiar and very nasty: French materialism, irreligion and Jacobinism dressed up in "crude notions", arrived at by either a simple misunderstanding of the nature of life or devised with some more sinister intent.

For James Jackson senior, a Boston physician, writing on the Brunonian system in 1809, its essential features seemed to be of a rather different sort. In the early nineteenth century, educated Boston physicians saw themselves as the source of light in a country of medical darkness. Hostile to systematizing of all kinds, they portrayed themselves as the custodians of cautious, empirical, and sceptical medicine. They identified medical progress with the clinics of London and Paris, and with the gradual accumulation of knowledge by means of the bedside description of disease and the labours of the post-mortem room.[85] Thus on the very first page of his account of Brunonianism, Jackson wrote that, at a time "when the wisest physicans had already entered the path of truth, that of observation, experience and induction; the path which Hippocrates and Sydenham had trod with so much success; and at a period when all were desirous to follow in this path ... Brown ... declared, that by the discovery of one principle he was able to explain all the secrets of physiology and medicine." In so doing, he "imitated all theorists in distorting all the other phenomena of nature".[86] Jackson saw as the essence of Brunonianism its methodological prescriptions which contained an idea "directly in opposition" to "the science of medicine".[87] "According to Brown," Jackson wrote, "it is useless to record the phenomena of disease, to collate and compare cases; for these phenomena, these symptoms, are fallacious."[88] All this, he wrote, was contrary to "the plan of observation and experience ... by which some men in all ages have been qualified to render more or less service to the sick, in spite of the various systems which the fashions of various ages have rendered popular."[89]

Thus a single medical principle was both the keystone and the fundamental flaw in Brunonianism. Excitability was nothing more than a speculative hypothesis, "the properties [of living things] . . . are discoverable only by observation and experiment."[90] The dangers of Brunonianism were all too obvious: it was simple, whereas experience taught that medicine was complex. It indulged indolence and discouraged medical men "from poring over the observations of others".[91] Systematizing had led Brown to egregious errors. It was possible to conclude from Brown's system that "there cannot be any such thing as a strictly local disease." This, Jackson said, was "stargazing".[92] Jackson, a man trained in London and Paris hospital medicine, was, of course, highly sympathetic to the idea that all diseases were local.

It is hardly surprising to find such a reading of Brown in this Boston physician. For him, the essence of Brunonianism was its method, the erection of a system of medicine on philosophical principles. Here, at least, Jackson was in agreement with the author of

[85] See Warner, op. cit., note 56 above, pp. 11–36.
[86] James Jackson, *Remarks on the Brunonian system,* Boston, Thomas B. Wait, 1809, pp. vii–viii.
[87] Ibid., p. ix.
[88] Ibid., p. viii.
[89] Ibid., p. ix.
[90] Ibid., p. 6.
[91] Ibid., p. 48.
[92] Ibid., pp. 45–6.

the *Inquiry*. But if for Brown this was a triumph, for Jackson it was a disaster. Systems of any sort denied the value of experience and learning, and appealed only to the simplifiers and the simple. To embattled Boston physicians, aristocrats of the American medical world, who had staked their claim on scepticism, nosography, post-mortem and tradition, Brunonianism posed the threat of democracy and equality among medical practitioners. It was the sort of medicine that gave legitimacy to quacks, herbalists, homeopaths, Perkinistic practitioners, electricians, Mesmerists and the whole tribe of toadstool millionaires.[93]

If Thomas Beddoes had seen Brown's system as essentially different from Cullen's, John Thomson saw it as essentially the same, a downright plagiarism in fact. Thomson was an Edinburgh-trained surgeon who had been a student when Cullen was an old man. Later, when Thomson became an extramural teacher of surgery in Edinburgh, he was committed to the view that surgery and physic were the practical faces of one basic discipline, pathology. It was a position which he defended in numerous publications. His biography of Cullen and his edition of Cullen's works were also enterprises devoted to demonstrating this.[94] The élitism of physicians, which was how Thomson represented Brunonianism, was anathema to him. In situating Brown and Cullen, Thomson reconciled apparently opposite propositions. On the one hand, he represented Brown's system as that of a simpleton, and Cullen's work as that of a profound and original thinker; and, on the other, he portrayed Brown as having stolen the principles of his system from Cullen. In his account of Brunonianism Thomson also discussed Beddoes's interpretation of Cullen.

There was nothing new in Brown's thinking, Thomson protested. The appeal of his opinions lay only in the "novelty of the terms . . . the simplicity of the views . . . and the ease with which a knowledge of these could be attained".[95] Unlike the radical Beddoes, but like the Tory Morrison, Thomson took the view that Brown had "attributed the phenomena of the animal economy to the agency of a single unknown principle".[96] Moreover, also like Morrison, he argued that Brown was not the first to do so. Brown's excitability, he said, "comprehends nothing more than what had been expressed by preceding physiologists and pathologists under the various appellations of Soul, Sentient Faculty, Archeus, Vitality or Vital Principle, and Animal Power, or Energy of the Brain."[97] Cullen himself, Thomson added, had used the terms "Excitability", "Exciting Powers", and "Excitement". Thomson then addressed Beddoes's mechanistic reading of Cullen, and cited Cullen to the following effect: "We suppose", said Cullen, animal "life, so far as it is corporeal, to consist in the excitement of the nervous system".[98] This, said Thomson, was not a simple mechanist statement of the Boerhaaveian sort, as Beddoes suggested, but a new idea of vitality, of which Brown had presented a derivative version. Similarly, Thomson claimed, the opinion that life was a forced state was one that "Dr Brown must have had repeated opportunities of

---

[93] James Harvey Young, *The toadstool millionaires,* Princeton University Press, 1961.

[94] I have discussed the social and intellectual context of Thomson's views in Christopher Lawrence, 'The Edinburgh Medical School and the end of the "Old Thing" ', *Hist. Universities,* 1988, **7**: 259–86.

[95] Thomson, op. cit., note 15 above, p. 224.

[96] Ibid., p. 228.

[97] Ibid., p. 229.

[98] Ibid., p. 230.

hearing" from Cullen.[99] In addition, Thomson claimed, this view could be found in Cullen's printed *Materia medica*. This, said Thomson, was the meaning of the following sentence from Cullen:

> That the soul is constantly necessary to the motion of the body we readily admit, but the argument is pushed too far, when it is supposed that these motions are supported by the power of the soul alone; for it appears that motions, excited by the impulse of external bodies, are absolutely necessary to that support.[100]

"In . . . considering the nervous system as the seat of his excitability", Thomson continued, "Dr Brown's opinions . . . were derived from, or modelled upon, those of his preceptor."[101] This, Thomson averred, was the import of Cullen's sentence, "The power of excitement . . . distinguishes the vital solid . . . but the brain, as uniting the whole nervous system has peculiar functions upon which the rest is dependent."[102] However, although Thomson represented Brown as having taken the idea of a single vital principle in the nervous system from Cullen, Thomson was equally concerned to show that Cullen, unlike Brown, *really* believed in three vital powers. Cullen, Thomson wrote, was "at great pains to distinguish between the sentient power or irritability of the nervous fibres,—the moving power . . . of the muscular fibres,—and the animal or innervatory power or energy of the brain."[103] Only once, said Thomson, did Cullen "somewhat unguardedly" comprehend the three powers under one common term.[104] It was this unguarded moment which was the source of Brown's idea of a *single* vital power: excitability.

Why was Thomson at such pains to represent Cullen as having really posited three vital principles, which Brown stole and conflated into one? Brown, said Thomson, by using only one principle could draw the conclusion that "sense, motion, the mental functions, and the passions, . . . are all produced . . . by mechanical impulse."[105] Thomson, in other words, accused Brown of using only one principle since he believed mental and corporeal functions to be identical. He was, in other words, a materialist. It was for this reason that Thomson represented Cullen as the teacher of three vital principles, one of which was the origin of mental operations. Thomson, the Whig, member of the Edinburgh establishment, former pupil and friend of Dugald Stewart, was imputing stout religious orthodoxy to the Edinburgh professoriate. Thomson's biography contains no suggestion that Cullen was a materialist. Accusations of this sort, however, had been bandied about in earlier years.[106] What Thomson saw as central to Brown's system was the abuse of an unguarded remark by a great professor.

In a later passage, Thomson performed an almost identical piece of surgery on the texts. Once again he identified Brown as a materialist, excused Cullen from such an

[99] Ibid., p. 231.
[100] Ibid., p. 232.
[101] Ibid., p. 237.
[102] Ibid., p. 239.
[103] Ibid., p. 238.
[104] Ibid., p. 239.
[105] Ibid., p. 240.
[106] Of Cullen's account of the nervous system Alexander Bower reflected, "His theories on this subject combined the most palpable materialism which was ever delivered". *A history of the University of Edinburgh*, Edinburgh, Alex. Smellie, 1817, vol. 1, p. 387.

accusation, and simultaneously pointed to plagiarism on Brown's part. Brown's view, said Thomson, quoting him, was that all stimuli act by "evident impulse".[107] Thomson argued that Brown had pilfered the idea from Cullen, who, in another unguarded moment no doubt, "seems to have taken [it] incautiously from Mr Locke."[108] Brown stole the idea from the following passage of Cullen's: "we know" wrote Cullen "of no other action of bodies on each other but that of impulse."[109] Such a passage, however, being open to misconstruction as materialist, Thomson added that Dr Cullen "seems to have been aware that the supposition of the phenomena of living systems, being produced by the operation of impulse alone, is founded upon a partial consideration of these phenomena."[110] Thomson then quoted the appropriate passage to prove that Cullen really did not believe "an hypothesis which . . . [explains] all the actions produced in the animal economy by mechanical impulse."[111]

And so Thomson went on, demonstrating Brown's plagiarism by juxtaposing passages from his works with passages from Cullen which meant, Thomson said, exactly the same thing. For instance, Brown's assertion that "Predisposition to disease is a middle state of Excitement between perfect health and disease", was, Thomson averred, identical to Cullen's view "that health may deviate, on either side, from the standard without passing to the opposite state, that of disease."[112] Similarly, Brown's distinction between direct debility and indirect debility was recognized by Cullen in his account of "repeated excitement . . . wearing out the system", and his statement that "such is the constitution of the nervous system that every unusual degree of excitement is followed by a proportional degree of collapse."[113] There remained for Brown, said Thomson, "only the merit of having applied the term[s]".[114]

There was, however, one area in which Thomson represented Brown's system as quite unlike that of Cullen's. Brown, according to Thomson, supposed that all the "morbid conditions of the different organs and functions" could be reduced to "two opposite conditions of the animal economy".[115] Cullen by contrast, Thomson said, had taught a complex pathological doctrine based on the concept of a variety of possible proximate causes. The reasons for Thomson's reading of the texts in this fashion relate to his occupation as a surgeon and his interest in general pathology. By the early nineteenth century, the surgeons in Edinburgh had eroded much of the power of the physicians, and in doing so they had gained entry into the traditional areas of practice claimed by them. This collapse of the old order was both institutional and intellectual. Thomson, in his *Lectures on inflammation* of 1813, claimed that distinctions between medicine and surgery were spurious, since the distinction between their objects of study—external and internal diseases or local and general disorders— was based on a misunderstanding of disease processes, a fact made clear by clinical

---

[107] Thomson, op. cit., note 15 above, pp. 245–6.
[108] Ibid., p. 247.
[109] Ibid.
[110] Ibid.
[111] Ibid.
[112] Ibid., p. 253.
[113] Ibid., p. 255.
[114] Ibid., p. 256.
[115] Ibid., p. 259.

medicine and general pathology.[116] Pathology for Thomson was the fundamental medical science, based, as he conceived it, on experiment and post-mortem. It was a complex, hard and learned discipline, which underlay both medicine and surgery. It was a science which Thomson identified with Cullen's injunction to discover proximate causes.[117] Thus Thomson represented the Brunonian system as embodying everything that proper pathological science was not. Brunonianism was facile, easily apprehended, taught that there were only two pathological states, trivialized the importance of local disease, misunderstood the role of nosology and minimized the need for surgery by an insistence on the general nature of all disorders.

According to Thomson, the Brunonian practitioner had only a few simple decisions to make, the first being to decide whether disease was local or general. This was a distinction Thomson found entirely spurious: "how little foundation", he wrote, "there exists in nature for making so strict a division of diseases."[118] Thomson further noted that, although Cullen's nosology contained the classes of local and general diseases, Cullen "seems to have been at all times fully aware how often these two kinds of disease coexist."[119] This was, of course, a pathological doctrine central to Thomson's bid to unite medicine and surgery. Local and general disease were the objects of study of the same discipline, pathology, and the focus of clinical attention for physician and surgeon alike. But it was Brown's view, he said, quoting him, that local and general disease "differ in every essential respect".[120] Thomson's reading of Brown as hostile to the concept of local disease went further than this, however. According to Thomson, Brown had removed a whole class of local diseases, the inflammations, from the provenance of the surgeon, and stated they were a consequence of general dysfunction and thus properly within the sphere of the physician. Thomson then noted that perusal of Cullen's *First lines* would "leave but little doubt as to the source from which Dr Brown's opinion . . . had been derived".[121] This, however, was a reading of Brown similar to the one which imputed materialism to him. On the one hand, Thomson showed that Brown's views were mischievously derived from Cullen; and then he demonstrated that Cullen, like himself, actually held a rather different opinion. In this case, Thomson suggested that Cullen provided a far more sophisticated account of the relation of local to general disease which did not, in fact, privilege general disease over local.

Thomson then went on to give an account of the Brunonian practitioner's role after he had decided that a disease was a general disturbance. According to Thomson, the Brunonian practitioner had then only to discover whether the disorder was one of vigour or debility. Once again, Thomson attempted to rob Brown of invention by remarking that the two states "had been fully recognised and described [by Cullen] under the various terms of Increased and Diminished Action, Excitement and

[116] John Thomson, *Lectures on inflammation*, Edinburgh, William Blackwood, 1813. For a discussion of the breakdown of the boundaries between physic and surgery in Edinburgh and a guide to the literature see Lawrence, op. cit., note 94 above.

[117] Thomson, op. cit., note 15 above, p. 259.

[118] Ibid., p. 300.

[119] Ibid.

[120] Ibid.

[121] Ibid., p. 303.

Collapse, Reaction and Debility."[122] Brown, however, had gone too far and attempted "to refer all diseases to one or other of these two states, and to reduce the whole of medical practice to two general plans of treatment".[123]

Beddoes, in his estimate of Brown's work, had endorsed Brown's view that much of his originality lay in his recognition that reasoning to causes because of nosological similarity was fallacious. According to Brown, nosology was a misguided enterprise since two diseases, juxtaposed on a nosological table, might in fact originate in fundamentally different states of excitement. Thomson, however, identified this so-called insight of Brown's as a part of a fundamental failure to understand the aim of nosology. Thomson, who obviously thought that Brown had taken leave of his senses, wrote, "In his recommendation to physicians to judge of the . . . character of diseases by the nature of the exciting powers which produce or remove them, and not by the symptoms they exhibit . . ., Dr Brown seems to have lost sight altogether of the . . . principle . . . that all that can be known of [these exciting powers] . . . must be derived from the observation of the sensible effects":[124] in other words, the symptoms. Brown had thus completely confused symptomology, which is the art of judging vigour and debility by particular symptoms, with nosology, the expression in accurate characters of "the order which nature general observes . . . the concourse or succession of symptoms".[125] So risible, indeed, was Brown's reasoning, argued Thomson, that he had had to make use of nosology whether he liked it or not. Not surprisingly, Thomson continued, the nosology Brown implicity used was Cullen's. The putative vanquishing of nosology achieved by Brown and applauded by Beddoes produced a hostile response from Thomson, a surgeon and pathologist sympathetic to the new approach of grounding natural histories in morbid anatomy.

For Thomson, Brown's speculations "had their origin in personal spite, arising out of wounded vanity". In turn "the malignant and rancorous animosity displayed in the writings . . . take away the pleasure which might have been derived from the manifestation of such talent as he had evinced."[126] For Thomson, Brown's system was derived in its essentials from Cullen or, as in the case of the use of stimulants, "in a desire to contradict precepts inculcated by Dr Cullen in his lectures and writings".[127] All else was dross, jargon and neologisms, or worthless and dangerous prescription. It was a materialist system, void of surgical or pathological value. Thomson's perceptions of the proper nature of the theory and practice of medicine, with all that they entailed for the ordering of society, were those which were valued by the Edinburgh establishment. In 1831 he was made the first professor of pathology in the University.

Thomson, however, did not dispose of Brunonianism for good. In the nineteenth century a number of authors came to Brown's defence. One of these was the English physician, Benjamin Ward Richardson, whose biographical history of medicine,

[122] Ibid., p. 306.
[123] Ibid.
[124] Ibid., p. 308.
[125] Ibid.
[126] Ibid., p. 351.
[127] Ibid., p. 324.

Disciples of Aesclepius, included a short account of him. Richardson wrote: "In this purely mechanical day, when nothing is allowed that is not experimentally illustrated, the hypothesis of Brown may seem, and, I doubt not, does seem, a mere fancy."[128] Yet, for Richardson, there was something in Brown's work that showed its author "was a man gifted with curious insight, a man of genius of a very high order".[129] This genius lay in Brown's "abstract reading of vital phenomena".[130] For Morrison and Thomson, Brown had been a materialist and had utterly misconstrued the problem of life. For Richardson the reverse was the case. He wrote "To this day we have not come much nearer to the solution of the great question of life than the hypothetical solution which he [Brown] advanced."[131] For, said Richardson,

> his conception that every living thing is pervaded with some inherent quality or substance which is its natural portion, its allotted portion, and upon the stock of which its capability for life, long or short, depends, is as sound a view as has ever been advanced and explains more of the phenomena of life than any other.[132]

This, said Richardson, is what John Hunter called the vital principle. Richardson was himself a vitalist. "We may have to admit", he wrote, "that there is a quality or substance . . . which whether it be from the first allotted, or whether it be regularly replenished, endows every living thing with life."[133] Why then did Richardson construe Brown as holding the same view as himself rather than portray him as a materialist, as had more often been the case?

Richardson was in many respects the archetypal cultured Victorian doctor. From a relatively humble beginning he achieved great success. He was a gentleman (knighted indeed), broadly learned and a lover of history and the classics. He was also a devout man in an age in which the biological sciences, which for him evidenced the existence of a Deity, were—in T. H. Huxley's evolutionism or Michael Foster's experimental physiology—threatening a new materialism. Richardson's vitalism was part of his theology. Richardson believed in a supreme being, and held medicine to be one of the oldest and most humane arts, devoted to the relief of suffering. In reading Brown as a vitalist, he was creating a single, ageless medical profession and attributing to it Victorian conceptions of humanity and piety. For him the greatest profession could not be, since its historical beginning, anything other than learned and pious. As he put it in another context, "No medical man can be a materialist."[134] John Brown testified to that. With Richardson the cycle had come almost full circle. Brown the reformer, then the revolutionary, had become a conservative.

In other contexts, however, other readings remained possible. In America Brunonianism could still be made to stand, symbolically, as a threat. Competition from sectarians remained vigorous in American medicine well into the twentieth

[128] Richardson, op. cit., note 2 above, p. 253.
[129] Ibid.
[130] Ibid.
[131] Ibid.
[132] Ibid.
[133] Ibid., p. 254.
[134] Quoted in Sir Arthur Salusbury MacNalty, *A biography of Sir Benjamin Ward Richardson,* London, Harvey Blythe, 1950, p. 76.

century. By this time, however, the ideological defence of orthodoxy on the basis of observation and experience, employed by Jackson, had shifted to an appeal to the experimental and laboratory sciences as the agencies which conferred on the profession its right to be the legitimate guardian of the public's medical welfare.[135] In 1911, Richard Cole Newton MD published an address he had given to the Orange Mountain Medical Society on Brown and the Brunonian system. Newton quoted extensively from Richardson's account of Brown's work and summed up the significance of Brunonianism as follows:

> That a rational man should not only have attempted to build up, but actually did build up a theory of the etiology of all human diseases and their treatment upon such facts, which no one disputes, as that alcohol and opium, if taken in sufficient quantities, will allay pain and stimulate the imagination, would be quite incredible did not every student of the history of medicine know that the various systems and sects in the practice of medicine have been built up and defended on even more ephemeral grounds than these.[136]

The significance of Brunonianism lay not in its detail, but in the fact that it was a system built, like all systems, on random, uncontrolled, unscientific observation. Because it was a system, it assumed, said Newton, that "the physician not nature cures the disease."[137] Such theories and systems, he said, "form a refuge for the unlearned and narrow medical mind."[138] Further, they "can fool the laity and even arouse the wild enthusiasm of the prejudicial and unthinking practitioner."[139] But such "fiat medicine" was not "real medicine".[140] Sadly, he noted, some of Brown's ideas "are still exceedingly potent in the minds not only of the laity, but of the profession."[141] One of these "errors" was (and here Newton agreed with Richardson's reading but disagreed with the endorsement) that a "vital principle, vital energy or strength" is assigned to every being.[142] Such vitalism was nonsense, "a fundamental and foolish error which is one of the main props of fiat medicine".[143] Progress in medical science, however, was exposing such things for what they were. For instance

> the consumption of alcoholic beverages, the sheet-anchor of his system, has been steadily decreasing since Brown's day, and this decrease has been notable during the past few years, largely because the white light of science has been turned upon the study of the effects of alcohol upon the human body.[144]

Everywhere, Newton observed, systems, or "fiat medicine", were falling prey to "scientific investigation".[145] He concluded:

---

[135] See Warner, op. cit., note 56 above.

[136] Richard Cole Newton, 'John Brown M.D. and the Brunonian system of medicine', *Medical Record,* 2 December 1911, pp. 1–23.

[137] Ibid., p. 20.

[138] Ibid., p. 22.

[139] Ibid., p. 23.

[140] Ibid.

[141] Ibid., p. 18.

[142] Ibid., p. 19.

[143] Ibid., p. 20.

[144] Ibid., p. 18.

[145] Ibid., p. 19.

We still have doctrines and systems and hypothetical explanations of natural phenomena, but the white light of science has grown too strong for us. The medicine of the future will, we believe, not be, like that of the past, largely controlled by dogma, superstition and tradition. It will be scientific medicine and the true physician of the future will not be ashamed to say that he does not know a thing that science has not yet made clear to him, and will not condemn an innovation simply because it does not conform to his theories, and because he cannot measure it with his yardstick.[146]

Newton's account is the one that might be expected from a learned American MD at this time. The essence of Brunonianism was its systematic construction; it was read by this American physician as an object lesson on the evils of populism and the necessity of making experimental science the cornerstone of practice.

My intention in presenting these differing accounts of Brown's career and the career of his writings should now be sufficiently plain. Scrutiny of previous readings of Brown's texts reveals that authors could not agree on their essential meanings; or, put another way, different readers have discerned different essential meanings according to their situation. Even excitability, apparently a key feature of the system, was represented differently by Beddoes and Morrison. Recently historians have begun to turn their attention to these sorts of questions, to study, for example, not the works and influence of some essential John Hunter, but a number of rather different John Hunters made for a specific purpose by subsequent generations, and in turn handed on to us as an apparently uncomplicated object, the father of scientific surgery.[147] Similarly, historians have now found that there was not one Newton in the eighteenth century, but many.[148] The discovery that, from day one, Brown's texts were the subject of interpretation does not mean that the modern historian can now return to them and gain privileged access to some putative essential meaning; quite the reverse. It should free the historian from the constraint of having to discover the meanings Brown's texts have for us, and lead to an understanding of the place of Brown and his work in the eighteenth and nineteenth centuries.

[146] Ibid., p. 23.

[147] See L. S. Jacyna, 'Images of John Hunter in the nineteenth century', *Hist. Sci.*, 1983, **21**: 85–108. See also P. B. Wood, 'The hagiography of common sense: Dugald Stewart's account of life and writings of Thomas Reid', in A. J. Holland (editor), *Philosophy, its history and historiography*, Dordrecht, D. Reidel, 1983, pp. 305–22. See Wood's first footnote for similar material dealing with French doctors and natural philosophers. See also J. R. R. Christie, 'Joseph Black and John Robison', in A. D. C. Simpson (editor), *Joseph Black 1728–1799. A commemorative symposium*, Edinburgh, The Royal Scottish Museum, 1982, p. 47–52.

[148] Simon Schaffer, 'Natural philosophy', in G. S. Rousseau and Roy Porter (editors), *The ferment of knowledge*, Cambridge University Press, 1980, pp. 55–92.

Medical History, Supplement No. 8, 1988, 22–45.

BRUNONIANISM UNDER THE BED: AN ALTERNATIVE TO UNIVERSITY MEDICINE IN EDINBURGH IN THE 1780s

by

MICHAEL BARFOOT*

'. . . They agreed with me that it looked serious; but they both strongly dissented from the view I took of the treatment. We differed entirely in the conclusions which we drew from the patient's pulse. The two doctors, arguing from the rapidity of the beat, declared that a lowering treatment was the only treatment to be adopted. On my side, I admitted the rapidity of the pulse, but I also pointed to the alarming feebleness as indicating an exhausted condition of the system, and as showing a plain necessity for the administration of stimulants. The two doctors were for keeping him on gruel, lemonade, barley-water, and so on. I was for giving him champagne, or brandy, ammonia and quinine. A serious difference of opinion, as you see! a difference between two physicians of established local repute, and a stranger who was only an assistant in the house. For the first few days, I had no choice but to give way to my elders and betters; the patient steadily sinking all the time. I made a second attempt to appeal to the plain, undeniably plain, evidence of the pulse. Its rapidity was unchecked, and its feebleness had increased. The two doctors took offence at my obstinacy. They said, "Mr Jennings, either we manage this case, or you manage it. Which is it to be?" I said, "Gentlemen, give me five minutes to consider, and that plain question shall have a plain reply." When the time expired, I was ready with my answer. I said, "You positively refuse to try the stimulant treatment?" They refused in so many words. "I mean to try it at once, gentlemen."—"Try it, Mr Jennings; and we withdraw from the case." I sent down to the cellar for a bottle of champagne; and I administered half a tumbler-full of it to the patient with my own hand. The two physicians took up their hats in silence, and left the house.'

The disease referred to in this passage was a fever. The conflict about how to cure it is instantly recognizable to historians of medicine familiar with the life and works of John Brown.[1] The essentials of the conflict between Brunonians and orthodox eighteenth-century practitioners are represented here. Where one saw an exhausted system which required stimulation, to the other it was a phlogistic diathesis which required sedative remedies. The details about the social milieu also seem correct. Mr Jennings, the crypto-Brunonian, was a stranger and had the lowly status of an assistant. His adversaries were physicians of reputation; they outnumbered him. The consultation eventually broke down acrimoniously.

In fact the extract is taken from *The moonstone* by Wilkie Collins, first published in 1868.[2] In his preface, the novelist prided himself on the accuracy of the medical details which play such a crucial role in the narrative; and there is no reason to doubt that they

* Michael Barfoot, PhD, Archivist, Lothian Health Board, Medical Archive Centre, Edinburgh University Library, George Sq., Edinburgh EH8 9LJ.

[1] See *The works of Dr John Brown, to which is prefixed a biographical account of the author by William Cullen Brown, M.D.*, 3 vols., London, J. Johnson, 1804. See also G. B. Risse, 'The Brownian system of medicine: its theoretical and practical implications', *Clio Medica*, 1970, **5**: 45–51; and *idem*, 'The history of John Brown's medical system in Germany during the years 1790–1806', Ph.D. diss., University of Chicago, 1971, pp. 68–135.

[2] See Wilkie Collins, *The moonstone* (1868), edited by J. I. M. Stewart, Harmondsworth, Penguin Books, 1966, p. 421.

reflect the climate of medical opinion as it stood in England during the mid-nineteenth century. This raises the question of whether the views of medical men, who thought and practised in a manner similar to the fictional Mr Jennings, can be ascribed to the influence of John Brown and the Brunonian system of medicine?

In 1809, when Bartholomew Parr published his article on fever, inflammation, and phlebotomy for the *London medical dictionary*, it seemed to him that medical practice was undergoing a significant and profound change.[3] Parr doubted the efficacy of bleeding in cases of certain fevers and other diseases where it had always been indicated. He made it quite clear that there had been a shift of sensibility about bleeding in order to alleviate phlogistic diatheses. Inflammation was interpreted more and more as an indication of debility rather than excitement. Its cure therefore required forms of stimulation, rather than such sedative remedies as blood-letting. Received wisdom throughout most of the eighteenth century was that theories might come and go, but practice remained the same. In particular, the dominant antiphlogistic regimen of bleeding, purging, blistering, sweating, and vomiting was the standard way of treating diseases considered phlogistic or inflammatory. There had always been exceptions where bleeding was prohibited—even in phlogistic, or sthenic diseases, as they also came to be known. So where had this apparent change of practice come from?

Parr could not give a satisfactory answer. He tentatively suggested that the interpretation of inflammation as debility, rather than excitement, originated among the private teachers at Edinburgh, rather than the University professors.[4] The significant point, however, is that he did not give any credit to Brown for inaugurating the new form of restorative practice. In fact, he gave the opposite impression by categorizing Brown as an old-fashioned bleeder:

> Brown was led to violent indiscriminate bleeding in his revival of the Methodic system, and he could not discover his error, as he had little experience. His pupils have unfortunately not always been enlightened by their errors.[5]

Other commentators disagreed. Charles Maclean, a lecturer for the East India Company on diseases in hot climates, shared the view that medical practice had been transformed. Looking back from the early 1820s, he spoke of "the immensity of the change which ha[d] taken place in the practice of physic".[6] Maclean claimed much of

---

[3] Bartholomew Parr, *The London medical dictionary*, 3 vols., London, J. Johnson and others, 1809, vol. 1, 642–55; vol. 2, pp. 13–25; 385–91.

[4] Ibid., p. 13. The names Parr mentioned were a Dr Lubbock and John Allen, a lecturer in physiology from the extramural school. His authority for this statement was based on A. Philips Wilson, *A treatise on febrile diseases, including intermitting, remitting, and continued fevers, eruptive fevers; inflammations; hemmorrhagies; and profluvia; in which an attempt is made to present, whatever, in the present state of medicine it is requisite for the physician to know respecting the symptoms, causes and cures of those diseases*, 4 vols., Winchester, J. A. Robbins, 1799–1804, vol. 3, p. 25. Wilson was himself an Edinburgh extramural medical lecturer. See vol. 1, pp. 490–533, for Wilson's discussion of Brown's system which, while critical, also stated that when all the other systematists were forgotten, "there will remain enough of the Brunonian doctrines to preserve the memory of the author" (p. 490).

[5] Ibid., vol. 2, p. 387. Parr went even further in the article on the 'Brunonian system', vol. 1, pp. 284–7, where he stated that Brown had not even visited a sick bed.

[6] Charles Maclean, *Evils of quarantine laws and non-existence of pestilential contagion; deduced from the phenomena of the plague of the Levant, the yellow fever of Spain and the cholera morbus of Asia*, London, T. and G. Underwood and others, 1824, p. vii.

the credit for this himself, but he also acknowledged another source of innovation. His own research and experiments on epidemic diseases in Calcutta and the Levant

> were originally suggested by the new and luminous views of the philosophic author of the "Elementa Medicinae Brunonis"; whom less prejudiced posterity, I venture to predict, will not hesitate to acknowledge as the Hippocrates of the 18th century.[7]

This difference of opinion about Brown's influence can in part be related to the ways in which Parr and Maclean were trained. Parr completed his medical education in Edinburgh in 1773, some five years before Brown began to lecture extramurally.[8] Maclean was a student there just over a decade later in 1784, when Brown's impact was at its height.[9] His loyalty was probably typical of many of those who, during the course of acquiring a more formal education at the University, also attended Brown's lectures and heard the debates at the Medical Society.[10] However, others present in Edinburgh around the same time held views diametrically opposite to Maclean. They saw Brown as a plagiarist, a pale imitation of William Cullen, without his experience of practice.[11] Somewhere in between the Brunonians and anti-Brunonians was yet another group. Its adherents discussed, developed and disseminated ideas similar to those adopted by

[7] *Idem, Results of an investigation respecting epidemic and pestilential diseases, including researches into the Levant concerning the plague*, 2 vols., London, Thomas and George Underwood, 1817, p. 53. In his subsequent book, *Practical illustrations of the progress of medical improvement, for the last thirty years: or histories of cases of acute diseases, as fevers, dysentery, hepatitis, and plague, treated according to the principles of the doctrine of excitation*, London, printed for the author, 1818, pp. xxxvii–xxxix, Maclean stated that his only criticism of Brown was that he had retained a small category of diseases which were due to sthenia or the phlogistic diathesis. Nevertheless, Maclean continued to insist that Brown had done more to approximate medicine to science than perhaps any of his predecessors, and that "his fundamental position will for ever remain the foundation of medical science, or rather the science of life" (p. xxxix). See also William Yates and Charles Maclean, *A view of the science of life on the principles established in the 'Elements of medicine' of the late celebrated John Brown M.D.* [etc.], Calcutta, 1797.

[8] See University of Edinburgh, MS Da., Album Academiae ab Anno 1762, ad annum 1786. Parr attended the University for the 1769–70, 1770–71, and 1771–72 sessions, fulfilling the course requirements for the degree, which he obtained in 1773. He is not to be confused with Dr Samuel Parr, the noted Whig minister who was a family friend, and to whom William Cullen Brown dedicated his edition of his father's works.

[9] Maclean attended the University during the 1784–85, and 1785–86 sessions, and took courses in Anatomy, chemistry, the practice of medicine and "Nos. Reg", or nosology. Unfortunately, class lists for Brown's lectures have not survived.

[10] See James Grey, *History of the Royal Medical Society 1737–1937*, Edinburgh University Press, 1952, pp. 50–61. For an earlier account, see William Stroude, 'History of the Royal Medical Society', in *List of members, laws and library catalogue, of the Medical Society of Edinburgh, instituted 1737; incorporated by Royal Charter Dec. 14, 1778*, Edinburgh, William Aitken, 1820.

[11] For example, see John Thomson, *An account of the life, lectures, and writings of William Cullen, M.D., Professor of the Practice of Physic at the University of Edinburgh*, 2 vols., Edinburgh, William Blackwood and Sons, 1859, vol. 2, pp. 222–487. In his *Lectures on inflammation exhibiting a view of the general doctrines pathological and practical of medical surgery*, Edinburgh, James Ballantyne for William Blackwood and others, 1813, Thomson opposed accounts of inflammation in terms of debility. However, like Parr, he associated these with Lubbock and John Allen, not Brown. Lubbock was prominent in the Royal Medical Society when Brown's ideas were deeply controversial and the main topic of debate. See R. Lubbock, 'Are contagions producing idiopathic disease directly or indirectly, debilitating?', Royal Medical Society, MS Dissertations of the Medical Society, vol. 14, 1782–1783, pp. 55–69. John Allen was also active in the Society. See 'Case AB [of Mania]', in Glasgow University Library, MS Gen. 1476, Allen Thomson Papers, Box 24, pp. 1–26. With Thomson, he subsequently defended Hume's philosophy against James Gregory, the Professor of the Practice of Medicine. See 'A necessitarian', *Illustrations of Mr. Hume's essay concerning liberty and necessity in answer to Dr Gregory in Edinburgh*, London, J. Johnson, 1795. There is also a manuscript copy of Allen's lectures in Edinburgh University Library, MS Gen. 2007/6.

Brunonians, but were less generous than Maclean in giving Brown any credit. For example, Erasmus Darwin wrote:

> The coincidence of some parts of this work with correspondent deductions in the *BRUNONIAN ELEMENTA MEDICINAE*—a work (with some exceptions) of great genius—must be considered as a confirmation of the theory, as they were probably arrived at by different trains of reasoning.[12]

From a broader national perspective, even those who identified themselves as Brunonians or anti-Brunonians were probably just a tiny minority of the medical practitioners who responded to changes in theory and practice that were taking place. As the nineteenth century progressed, most medical men were never actually in a position either to acknowledge or repudiate Brown's role. They simply absorbed an approach which was by then widely diffused throughout the culture. A similar point was explicitly made by an article on Brunonianism in *The Edinburgh medical and physical dictionary* of 1807.[13] It began by noting that Brunonian language and sentiments had become such an established feature of medical culture in Scotland and elsewhere in the world that it was necessary to have a working knowledge of its principal tenets. Yet the "remarkable thing is that a majority of the persons who are become converts to the doctrine, are totally unable to recollect, when or how they were converted."[14] Thus, even if the fictitious Mr Jennings had been a real medical practitioner in Britain during the mid-nineteenth century, he may not have had the slightest idea about the history of the practices he adopted.

In view of this confusing situation, the currently accepted view that Brown's ideas had little impact in Britain, while it cannot be conclusively refuted, cannot be substantiated either.[15] Should one wish to proceed in the face of the divided testimony of medical men at the time, some basis must be found to decide who was "right" and who was "wrong" about the extent of Brunonian influence. Yet how is this to be

[12] Erasmus Darwin, *Zoonomia; or the laws of organic life*, 2 vols., London, J. Johnson, 1794–1796, vol. 1, p. 75. Darwin's claim to be a co-discoverer were widely commented on at the time, and considered to be less than ingenuous. For example, see Thomas Beddoes, *Observations on the nature and cure of calculus, sea scurvey, consumption, catarrh, and fever, together with conjectures upon several other subjects physiological and pathological*, London, J. Murray, 1793, footnote, pp. 160–1; *The English review; or an abstract of English and foreign literature*, 1795, **34**: 349–53. See also A. Philips Wilson, *An essay on the nature of fever, being an attempt to ascertain the principles of its treatment*, Worcester, J. Tymbs, 1807, pp. 46–88, 164. After discussing the laws of excitability of the animal system in the Medical Society, and lecturing on febrile diseases, Wilson subsequently became Physician to Worcester Infirmary. He accordingly regretted his earlier high estimation of Brunonianism: "I had conceived a strong prejudice in favour of it before I was capable of estimating its merits, and it was long before I could persuade myself that it had in fact made no real addition to our knowledge" (p. 164).

[13] *The Edinburgh medical and physical dictionary*, 2 vols., Edinburgh, Bell and Bradfute and others, 1807, vol. 1, s.v. 'Brunonianism or Brunonian system'.

[14] Ibid. Beddoes, op. cit., note 12 above, p. 160, also spoke of the widespread diffusion and secret influence of Brown's ideas upon practice. Even highly critical reviews acknowledged his genius and contribution to medicine. For example, see the *Analytical review, or history of literature, domestic and foreign*, 1789, **4**: 166–71, which stated that "the Doctrine" had made "a deep impression on those qualified to judge of its value; it had introduced into practice some important innovations, and these innovations are acknowledged and followed by many who refuse their assent to the principles of Dr Brown, or who have bestowed no pains in examining his opinions" (p. 166).

[15] See Grey, op. cit., note 10 above, p. 57; G. B. Risse, 'The quest for certainty in medicine: John Brown's system of medicine in France', *Bull. Hist. Med.,* 1971, **45**: 1–12, p. 2.

done? Any appeal to information in the accounts of Brown's life and opinions by Thomas Beddoes, William Cullen Brown, and John Thomson falls back into the same conflict of interpretation.[16] An alternative approach might be to claim Brown had no "real" influence because he never made an original contribution to medicine. However, it is doubtful whether an objective, rational case for Brown's plagiarism, based upon a comparison of Brown's and William Cullen's works, could actually be made.[17] Even if it were possible, this would only beg the question of whether Cullen was himself an innovative thinker. All this would succeed in doing is to recapitulate features of the historical debate itself. Where the Cullenians were dismissive, Brown's apologists could just as easily point to differences with Cullen's approach and defend Brown's originality.

Another strategy widely used to denounce Brown at the time was to attack his experience as a practical physican. Many besides Parr intimated that Brown had very little practice compared, for example, with Cullen; and that such practice as came his way, had been conducted badly.[18] In reply, Brunonians pointed out that Brown was prevented from practising in Edinburgh. They also defended his record and pointed to successful cures by his followers. Given the incommensurability between the contents of eighteenth-century and modern medical discourse, it is actually very difficult to evaluate whether Brown's practice was misguided and pernicious in comparison with that of Cullen or other figures. Yet unless one can show this, the argument carries no weight today. Certainly, there are many case histories of patients treated by Cullen and other Edinburgh professorial practitioners, whereas Brown's practice is inaccessible. However, even if one accepts the disease classifications, details of therapies, and cure claims contained in hospital and other records at face value, the care outcome cannot be assessed without major reinterpretations in line with current medical knowledge and experience. If the case for Brown's influence is dismissed because of errors in his views about the causes and treatment of disease, the accounts of many other medical men who currently enjoy a more respectable place in the history of medicine might also have to be treated in the same way. Thus an appeal to the standards of modern medicine would rapidly get out of hand, and the whole period would take on the appearance of a graveyard of rejected medical knowledge.

Instead of being drawn into ultimately indefensible statements about the originality, correctness, and wider British influence of Brunonianism, another

---

[16] See Thomas Beddoes, 'Observations on the character and writings of John Brown M.D.', in *The elements of medicine of John Brown M.D.*, new ed., 2 vols., London, J. Johnson, 1795, vol. 1, pp. xxxv–cii; William Cullen Brown, 'Life of Dr John Brown', in op. cit., note 1 above, vol. 1, pp. xix–ccxxxi; John Thomson, op. cit., note 11 above, vol. 2, appendix, pp. 710–18. See also National Library of Scotland MS 5173, Elizabeth Cullen Brown, 'Reminiscences concerning John Brown' (1838), fols. 1–13. Although Beddoes was attacked by Brown's children for his biography, he was ambivalent towards Brown and Brunonianism, rather than overtly hostile. For example, as well as expressing reservations about Brown the man, his edition had Darwin's comment about Brown printed on the title page.

[17] However, a comparison of Cullen's and Brown's views which took account of changes in different editions of their various works would be useful. For example, at present it is not possible to see precisely how their doctrines changed during the course of successive editions; nor is there any means of assessing the reliability of the edited version of the *First lines of the practice of physic* and *Elementa medicinae*.

[18] For example, see *Lexicon medicum or medical dictionary*, 5th ed., London, Longman and others, 1825, pp. 211–12.

approach will be followed here. Brunonianism is viewed as a medical movement with a very distinctive ideological character. The account of health and disease it advanced was originally inseparable from the social and political values attached to it as a form of alternative medicine which emerged in Edinburgh during the late 1770s and early 1780s. Examining Brunonianism in relation to its local social context reveals how it developed in opposition to the medical establishment which decried it. It also enables an assessment of the effect it had on the Edinburgh medical community to be presented in a manner which avoids many of the difficulties outlined above.

Brown's original followers were drawn from the men who attended his lectures in Edinburgh between 1778 and 1786. Many of them were members of the Royal Medical Society, and those that were not, could be taken in as guests to swell the ranks of the pro-Brown lobby. Unfortunately, there is no recent history of the Society upon which to base a prosopography of those who wrote dissertations and discussed case histories along Brunonian lines.[19] Nor are there any reliable figures of the numbers involved. One source suggests that over 200 annually adopted Brunonianism.[20] Even if this estimate represents a fifty per cent exaggeration, it still makes those about whom some details are known painfully few. Of course, not all of the early Brunonians had medical careers.[21] Among those that did, only a minority took MDs. Some, however, did become distinguished physicians in their own right. Yet a Brunonian dissertation for the Royal Medical Society will hardly serve as evidence for a life-long commitment to the movement. A former allegiance to Brown, rather like one to Hobbes or Hume before him, may have been something that had to be denied even in private. If so, admissions in print should be thought of as exceptions, rather than the criterion for assessing the degree of Brunonian influence.

For a variety of reasons, then, there is a paucity of reliable information from which to reconstruct the beliefs, values, and attitudes which made up the Brunonian ideology. Only one early follower was prepared to go on record as a Brunonian. This was Robert Jones, who published *An inquiry into the state of medicine, on the principles of inductive philosophy* at the height of Brown's influence in Edinburgh.[22]

---

[19] See J. R. R. Christie, 'Edinburgh medicine in the eighteenth century; the view from the students', *Bull. Soc. soc. Hist. Med.*, 1976, **33**: 311–18. For two recent general accounts of the Society, see L. Rosner, 'Students and apprentices: medical education at Edinburgh University, 1760–1810', Ph.D. diss., Johns Hopkins University 1985, pp. 258–327; C. J. Lawrence, 'Medicine as culture: Edinburgh and the Scottish Enlightenment', Ph.D. diss., University of London, 1984, pp. 200–17.

[20] Op. cit., note 13 above. The article also made the point that, among these were many army and navy physicians who disseminated Brunonianism over the whole medical world.

[21] See Robert James Mackintosh (editor), *Memoirs of the life of the Right Honourable Sir James Mackintosh*, 2 vols., London, Edward Moxon, 1835, vol. 1, pp. 23–6. Mackintosh stated that he became a Brunonian in 1784, while studying for his medical degree. Later, he became an MP and a distinguished Whig political writer. He was the author of a 'Dissertation second, exhibiting a general view of the progress of ethical philosophy, chiefly during the seventeenth and eighteenth centuries', in the *Encyclopaedia britannica*, 7th ed., Edinburgh, Adam and Charles Black, 1842, vol. 1, pp. 293–429. Elizabeth Cullen Brown, op. cit., note 16 above, recounted a conversation which took place between Dr Parr and James Mackintosh about collaborating on Brown's biography. Parr said Mackintosh would have to supply him with "the medical matter" if he undertook the project.

[22] Robert Jones, *An inquiry into the state of medicine, on the principles of inductive philosophy, with an appendix containing cases and observations*, Edinburgh, T. Longman and T. Cadell, London, C. Elliott, 1781. Subsequent references to Jones's *Inquiry* indicate this book. Jones's only other accredited work is *An inquiry into the nature, causes and termination of nervous fevers; together with observations tending to*

Next to nothing is known of Jones's life. However, his narrative provides ample compensation for this. Jones gave a direct and passionate view of the Edinburgh medical community, one which discarded many of the eighteenth-century conventions of literary politeness and actually named names.[23] Although his exposé emerged from a very definite point of view, it was much more than a polemical rag. Jones made it quite clear that his attack was upon a group of men, rather than the personalities of individual professors; and, on the whole, he maintained this stance. By way of a returned compliment, his views are treated here as representative of early Edinburgh Brunonianism.

Jones's manifesto used three interrelated themes to express the principal features of Brunonian ideology. He gave a conjectural history of the rise and progress of medicine as an art, which culminated in the advent of Brunonianism as the first manifestation of scientific medicine. He created a heroic biography of Brown, the sage who first healed himself and then applied his findings inductively to all forms of universal disease. Finally, he attacked the antiphlogistic basis of Edinburgh medical practice, and showed how Brunonian procedures conformed to the methodology of inductive philosophy.

MEDICINE AS CONJECTURAL HISTORY

Although the genre of conjectural history by no means originated in eighteenth-century Scotland, some of its most notable contributors could be found among the literati closely associated with the flowering of Edinburgh Enlightenment culture.[24] Conjectural history in its broadest sense incorporated accounts of the rise and progress of social and political institutions, such as government and law; and of beliefs and practices, such as religion and morality. However, it also dealt with the institutionalization of human knowledge. This was discussed in terms of the origins

---

illustrate the method of restoring His Majesty to health and of preventing relapses of his disease, Salisbury, Robinson, 1789. On Jones, see Alfredo Ilardi, 'La medicina secondo i principi della filosofia induttiva nel pensiero di Robert Jones', *25th Congr. naz. Stor. Med.*, Forli-Bologna, 1971, (1973), pp. 403–6. William Cullen Brown, op. cit., note 1 above, vol. 1, p. cxlvii, claimed his father was the author. The same point was made by Elizabeth Cullen Brown in her 'Reminiscences', op. cit., note 16 above, fol. 9. Whether this was true or not is irrelevant to the use made of the *Inquiry* here. However, features of this work, which have no exact parallel in Brown's writings, do seem to match Jones's studies in both arts and medicine, and his attendance at the Royal Infirmary.

[23] Most of the information about Brown's early followers actually comes from Jones's *Inquiry*. For example, John Wainman is reported to have converted his father to Brunonian therapies for the intermittent fevers which were common in their practice in the Lincolnshire Fens. Of others mentioned, such as Richard Scott Byam, Richard Codrington, and John Watson Howell, little is known beyond their names in the matriculation albums. Those who were identified as eminent physicians included Edward Stevens, James Campbell, William Yates, and James M'Donnell. Stevens became an eminent gastric physiologist in America. Campbell and Yates practised in India; and the latter collaborated with Maclean to produce an analysis of fever cases at the General Hospital at Calcutta. M'Donnell was one of the founders of the Belfast Fever Hospital. Samuel Lynch and Mr Christie, finally, were two other pupils. The former compiled the 'Table of excitement and excitability' also known as "the Brunonian biometer", included in subsequent editions of Brown's works. The latter explained Brown's doctrine of excitement in terms of a complex analogy based around fuel burning in a grate. See Beddoes, op. cit., note 16 above, pp. cxix–cxxxvii.

[24] For a recent reassessment of this tradition, see R. L. Emerson, 'Conjectural history and Scottish philosophers', in D. Johnson and L. Ovellette (editors), *Historical papers 1984 Communications historiques*, Ottawa, Canadian Historical Association, 1984, pp. 63–90.

and development of the arts and sciences. Jones also adopted this framework to identify the character of medicine and to provide an account of its historical development as a discipline.

The ways in which the terms "arts" and "sciences" were used suggests they had very general, not to say ambiguous, connotations. There were liberal and mechanical arts, as well as those of luxury. Arts could also be described as polite, rude, or refined, which often added further complexities. The sciences could include metaphysics, religion, politics, criticism, and morals as well as, for example, mathematics and natural philosophy. To group such diverse subjects together may seem like a simple mistake. However, what seems like a fundamental confusion of epistemic categories, is actually quite consistent from another viewpoint. In common with other eighteenth-century users of these terms, Jones understood the arts and sciences less in relation to the boundaries between disciplines, and more as shorthand descriptions of two different activities. "Science" referred to the process of observing nature, collecting facts, and assembling histories, in order to discover the relations and laws which governed the particular phenomena in question. An "art" resulted from the application of this scientifically acquired knowledge for definite ends. Thus, for Jones, medicine was the art of preserving health and curing disease; at the same time, it could only achieve this beneficial end if it was also a science.

Because Jones interpreted medicine as an activity performed by men with particular goals in mind, the way was open for an analysis of the cultural dynamics which had affected its historical development. He catalogued the rapid progress made by almost all the arts of his day which were concerned with men's safety, subsistence, accommodation, and ornament. These had all received encouragement from the development of commerce. The rise of the inductive philosophy and its application to different branches of knowledge had also engendered greater freedom of enquiry. Scrutiny of the principles of evidence had improved the art of legislation. Even such unlikely candidates for reform as moral philosophy, criticism, and *belles-lettres* had become progressive through a reorganization upon scientific principles. Yet, within this optimistic survey of social and intellectual accomplishments, the art of medicine alone was stationary. The reasons for this were complex and Jones discussed them at some length. However they all stemmed from the fact that

> the medical profession remains in the condition of an art deprived of its science to analize and improve it; as we cannot perceive the most faint appearance of the inductive philosophy of Bacon applied for that purpose, or Sir Isaac Newton's axioms of natural philosophy, which can be shown to be universal axioms of nature.[25]

From Jones's perspective, physicians had an inadequate conception of medicine. They lacked knowledge of the foundations and rules which underwrote the practice of their particular liberal art. The history of medicine from antiquity to the late eighteenth century illustrated the unreformed state of medicine as a "rude", and "conjectural art". In Jones's hands, history became a mirror for physicians which reflected back their failings and provided lessons for the future of medicine in a new Brunonian age.

[25] Jones, *Inquiry*, op. cit., note 22 above, p. 4.

It was a standard ploy for all advocates of the inductive philosophy to abhor system, theory, and hypothesis as the enemies of scientific improvement. What Jones contributed was an assessment of the wider social and political conditions which favoured the reformation of medicine along inductive lines. During the course of his medical education at the University of Edinburgh, Jones almost certainly heard other conjectural histories of the rise and progress of medicine. He attended the theory and practice classes of James Gregory and William Cullen, who each gave historical introductory lectures to their courses.[26] He may also have heard a similar approach to anatomy, although Alexander Monro *secundus* reduced this part of his father's original course, where the history of the subject was more thoroughly treated.[27] However, other features of Jones's presentation suggest that conjectural histories of medicine by the faculty were by no means his only exemplars.

When Jones came to Edinburgh, he was clearly out to get himself much more than a medical education. In 1781, the last year his name appears in the University matriculation roll, he also attended natural philosophy, logic, moral philosophy, and law of nations classes.[28] These were taught by John Robison, John Bruce, Adam Ferguson, and Allan Maconochie. Each professor stressed the role that inductive philosophy had played in reforming his particular discipline, and Jones drew heavily upon them all.[29] If Bacon and Newton were cast into the roles of man-midwives who attended the birth of the inductive method, then Robison, and Bruce in particular, were Jones's wise men, bringing news of the nativity to far-off disciplines.[30] Throughout his discussion, Jones showed a keen appreciation of the wider social and political circumstances which affected the development of knowledge:

> The arts and sciences, we shall hereafter have occasion to observe, have been found to be considerably affected by the spirit of political laws. In free states they are cherished; in despotic ones they languish; notwithstanding which, they are, as in the course of nature, found to be progressive.[31]

[26] Jones studied anatomy with Monro *secundus* and chemistry with Black during the 1778–79 session. In the following year, he repeated Monro's course and attended Gregory's on the theory and Cullen's on the practice of medicine.

[27] See Emerson, op. cit., note 24 above, p. 79, for a discussion of the use of history by Monro *primus*.

[28] In the same year he also studied botany and materia medica, and attended clinical lectures at the Infirmary.

[29] For Robinson see John Playfair, 'Biographical account of the late John Robison LL.D., F.R.S.E., and Professor of Natural Philosophy in the University of Edinburgh', *Trans. Roy. Soc. Edinb.*, 1815, 7: 495–540; for Bruce, see Alexander Grant, *The story of the University of Edinburgh*, 2 vols., London, Longmans and Green, 1888, vol. 2, pp. 330–1; for Ferguson, see R. B. Sher, *Church and university in the Scottish Enlightenment: the moderate literati of Edinburgh*, Princeton University Press, 1985, pp. 117–19; for Maconochie, see the *DNB*. See also Edinburgh University Library, Mic. M 1070–1071, Meadowbank Papers.

[30] After Bacon and Brown himself, Bruce was by far the most quoted author. Jones referred to Bruce's recently published *First principles of philosophy for the use of students*, Edinburgh, William Creech and T. Cadell, 1780. A slightly modified second edition appeared a year later. Eventually Bruce expanded what was originally only a brief précis of his lectures into a full text, but this was after Jones' work was published. See *idem, Elements of the science of ethics on the principles of natural philosophy*, London, A. Strahan and T. Cadell, 1786. Robinson also published *Outlines of mechanical philosophy, containing the heads of a course of lectures*, Edinburgh, William Creech, 1781. Jones and Brown both admired Robison, under whom they studied at different periods. However, Brown seems to have been a student of John Stevenson, the former Professor of Logic and Metaphysics, in 1770, and his name does not appear in the matriculation album after 1775. Bruce was not appointed joint professor with Stevenson until 1774.

[31] Jones, *Inquiry*, op. cit., note 22 above, p. vii.

Certainly, the interrelationship of human knowledge, culture and social institutions would have been emphasized by all the professors in the Arts Faculty. However, it is doubtful whether the strongly republican political sentiments which pervaded Jones's discussion were adopted from his professorial mentors.[32] When Jones connected the spirit of political laws with the development of the different branches of learning, he may well also have been drawing on Hume's influential *Essays,* especially 'Of the rise and progress of the arts and sciences', where almost all the credit for the cultural sponsorship of learning and polite attainments was ascribed to republican government.[33]

Despite the many injustices of British social institutions, Jones was confident, medicine could be improved and catch up with other subjects. If the inductive method championed by Newton and Bacon was fully adopted, men would acquire the "indispensable qualifications which should centre in the character of a physician, those of historian, philosopher and artist".[34] However, there were still formidable obstacles involving the nature of medical education which had to be overcome:

> But if graduates are to be only believers, bigots, or, to use the phrase, Tories in medicine, by a blind attachment or passive obedience, to systems; in that case we must give up all hope, that the healing art will have its science to simplify and explain it.[35]

For Jones, the institutional basis for medical systems was the corporation. Foremost among these in Edinburgh was the University.[36] Once a beacon of learning, it had now been taken over by professors who peddled old knowledge for profit. As a result, the original intention of universities to benefit the community had been corrupted. Despite good service in the past, they had degenerated into so many "interested corporations". This had led to bigotry in religion and prejudice in philosophy. The individual's power to make independent judgments had been lost and fewer men thought for themselves. But if the full implications of the inductive philosophy were realized, then, Jones wrote, "a great part of mankind would find themselves qualified not only for making improvements, but discoveries."[37] Jones repeatedly contrasted the republicanism of the individual medical improver with the despotism of the faculty. In this way, the whole notion of medical reform advocated by Brunonianism was always connected with more general issues of cultural and

---

[32] This cannot be entirely ruled out without further research. Young professors, like regents before them, often entertained radical political ideas, which were revised as they ascended to positions of authority and responsibility. Bruce and Maconochie would be interesting cases to pursue. They were among the original founders of the Speculative Society. Bruce became a close political associate of Henry Dundas and eventually an MP. Maconochie, under the title Lord Meadowbank, became an eminent judge at the Court of Session.

[33] David Hume, 'Of the rise and progress of the arts and sciences', in *Essays, moral and political* (1741–1742), 2 vols., 3rd ed., London, A. Miller and A. Kincaid, 1748, vol. 2, pp. 156–92.

[34] Jones, *Inquiry*, op. cit., note 22 above, p. 31.

[35] Ibid., p. vii. For a similar view, expressed by Dr John Richard Marlyn in a resignation speech at the Royal Medical Society, see Royal Medical Society, Minutes of the Medical Society, 12 February 1781.

[36] Jones, *Inquiry*, op. cit., note 22 above, pp. 173–85; 366–7.

[37] Ibid., p. 179.

social change.[38] The movement nurtured and developed themes associated with classical republican, country Whig, and radical groups: the right of the independent, free-thinking individual, ready to bear arms against tyranny, political or intellectual; the corruption of social institutions by patronage and favouritism; and finally, the prospect of an intellectual republic, in which the franchise of human judgement would be extended beyond its current sphere.[39]

HEROIC BIOGRAPHY AND MEDICAL INDUCTION

Jones's historical drama would have been anticlimactic without a hero to set the medical world to right. The story of Brown's discovery of the true physic and the reception he received from the Edinburgh medical community provided Jones with a plot within a plot. Using carefully selected scenes of conflict between Brown and the University, College, and Infirmary physicians who dominated the Edinburgh medical school, he created a medical morality play. In places, the style and the setting actually resembled Collins's characterization of Jennings.[40] However, unlike the novelist, dramatic impact was not the only effect for which he strived. Brown's personal trials and public tribulations were presented in a forceful manner which aimed to attract further converts to Brunonianism. The young medical students had all been educated to regard truth as something which operated involuntarily upon the mind, according to the degree of evidence. The necessity of belief each experienced at Brown's lectures was frequently contrasted with the absence of felt conviction when listening to Monro or Cullen. Following Brown and his "New Doctrine" offered students the uplifting experience of conversion, and the promise of medical improvement delivered to the world through their hands.[41]

Although Jones's conjectural history referred to social, economic, and political factors which had affected the progress of medicine, they were not his sole concerns. Intellectual causes which retarded the development of human understanding, such as a psychological propensity to adopt systems, and the search for ultimate facts, were important too. Individual genius was also considered to have played a significant role in the progress of the arts and sciences. Indeed, at times when society and its institutions were unfavourable to progress, all hope rested upon the talents of

---

[38] In particular, see Jones's account of the different forms of government and their advantages and disadvantages, op. cit., note 22 above, pp. 156–72.

[39] When such terms as "Whig", "Tory", "radical", and "republican" are used in relation to the eighteenth century, this raises the complicated question of the relationship between the varieties of political thought described in these ways and political action itself, considered in terms of government and opposition. For a general discussion, see Q. Skinner, 'Some problems in the analysis of political thought and action', *Polit. Theor.*, 1974, **2**: 277–303; and H. T. Dickinson, *Liberty and property: political ideology in eighteenth-century Britain*, London, Methuen, 1977, pp. 1–10.

[40] Jones went into great detail about the case of John Isaacson, over which Brunonians, Andrew Duncan, and Monro *secundus* clashed. See the *Inquiry*, op. cit., note 22 above, pp. 134–53. For a reply see Andrew Duncan, *A letter to Dr Robert Jones of Caermarthenshire, in answer to an account which he has published of the case of Mr John Braham Isaacson, student of medicine, and to the injurious aspersions which he has thrown out against the physicians who attended Mr Isaacson*, Edinburgh, C. Elliot, 1782.

[41] The dedication to Brown at the beginning of the *Inquiry* stated: "But the nature of truth is such, that it needs only to be known to beget conviction". See also Library of the Royal College of Physicians of Edinburgh MS, Edinburgh Medical Society, 1779–80, 'Mr Campbells Brunonianism'.

specially gifted men. Thus Brown was presented as the first to apply the model of inductive inquiry to medicine, and his view of the animal economy was held up as a new and scientific way of proceeding. Brown began with the simple phenomena of health; he then considered the powers which operated upon men in that state and next, deviations from the healthy state; and finally, he moved on to disease itself. The logical progression—from health, to predisposition, to idiopathic disease—was analogous to the pattern of investigation in other reformed sciences. They all showed the same orderly progression, from the simple to the complex. By attributing all disease to the variation in degrees of excitement, Jones claimed, Brown had also avoided a multiplicity of causes, and created a sound basis for the interpretation of medical facts. This philosophical arrangement of evidence then paved the way for laws of nature affecting the animal economy to be discovered.

Jones also legitimized the scientific claims of Brunonian medicine by correlating the steps which led to Brown's discovery of excitement with those which led Newton to universal gravitation.[42] He also added details about Brown's struggle with gout, and the failure of orthodox antiphlogistic medicine to cure it. Throughout Brown was portrayed as an independent free-thinking genius who first had to close all the medical textbooks "and seal each of them with seven seals, till he saw what he might make of his own thoughts."[43] The result of this process was the revelation that "the human machine was nothing in itself, but in constant and momentary dependence upon a number of powers, perfectly distinct from it, the operation of which was necessary to its existence."[44] Nor was the doctrine of excitement limited to the animal kingdom. It was one department of a broader science of living matter which resulted from the universal application of Newton's first rule of reasoning. Thus if the doctrine of excitement was properly applied to agriculture, then farming would also be leached of its errors and take its place alongside medicine as a reformed art.[45]

Appeals to Baconian induction and Newton's rules of reasoning like those entertained by Jones were commonplaces at the time. There was a widespread consensus about this means of legitimizing knowledge so that it acquired the proper scientific pedigree. Hume sought to reform moral philosophy and natural religion along these lines, and thinkers as diverse as Priestley and Reid attempted much the same thing, although they hoped for less controversial results.[46] Hence, the rhetoric

[42] Jones, *Inquiry*, op. cit., note 22 above, p. 92.

[43] What evidence we have about Brown himself suggests he also identified with intellectual dissent and free-thinking. Thomas Somerville, in *My own life and times, 1741–1814*, Edinburgh, Edmonston and Douglas, 1861, pp. 134–40, discussed Brown, with whom he was at school. In particular, Somerville emphasized Brown's general independence of mind and that Brown was a secret sceptic and admirer of Hume's philosophy. Robert Kerr, in *Memoirs of the life, writings and correspondence of William Smellie*, 2 vols., Edinburgh, John Anderson, 1811, vol. 2, p. 262, relates an anecdote involving Brown, and William Smellie and Gilbert Stewart, two other Edinburgh outsiders who had been passed over for university preferment. During a walk together, a conversation took place between Brown and a mason adding the finishing touches to Hume's tomb on Calton Hill. Brown inquired whether Hume, "the honest gentleman", would be able to get out of such a strong building at the Resurrection. The mason replied: "I have secured that point, sir, for I have put the key under the door."

[44] Jones, *Inquiry*, op. cit., note 22 above, p. 109.

[45] Ibid., pp. 88–90. Agriculture is an important but neglected theme in Brown's works.

[46] Jones understood Newton's original rules as general maxims about casual reasoning. The first emphasized the parsimony of causes; the second the connection between similar causes and effects; while

of induction was just as likely to be used by conservative medical professors at Edinburgh University as it was by Brunonian opponents like Jones. By itself then, this is not enough to distinguish the intellectual content of the movement. However, the consequences which followed from a Brunonian application of Newton's rules to the animal economy were more unusual in later eighteenth-century Scottish medicine. To a Brunonian, the uniformity of animate nature was no different from its inanimate counterpart. In both, there was a regular succession of causes and effects. Life was a "forced state", the product of the action of stimuli upon matter which possessed the property of excitability. Other medical authors who used a similar rhetoric of scientific method, such as Robert Whytt and James Gregory, reserved an exceptional status for the phenomena of life and refused to associate it with matter of any kind. Cullen was frequently suspected of being a materialist because of the role he gave to the nervous fluid as the medium of sensation. Yet he also made special appeals to the *vis medicatrix naturae* as an occult power residing in the living body, while at the same time professing to follow the inductive method.[47]

THE ATTACK ON EDINBURGH MEDICAL PRACTICE

The final test of the status of Brunonianism as a medical art, based on a scientific understanding of the animal economy, was not just the discovery of laws of nature. It was their application to the useful purposes of life.[48] In the case of the medical art, this was to preserve health and cure disease. Therefore Brunonian medicine had to represent itself as a successful form of practice. Because of the important role that professorial physicians played in Edinburgh medical education, it is rarely appreciated just how limited their own opportunities for actual practice could be. Most of the general practice in Edinburgh was in the hands of local surgeon-apothecaries.[49] The private practice which was available came from the aristocratic, gentry, and professional classes and was controlled by a small, very exclusive group of physicians. Alexander Monro *secundus* inherited the practice of his father, who had been a surgeon-apothecary. Robert Whytt and Joseph Black were helped by their international reputations. However, such outsiders as John Gregory and Cullen had to work hard to achieve a local success, despite their prominent positions in the medical school. Although teaching success was important, it probably was not

---

the third dealt with inferences from observed to unobserved causes. For a wider discussion, see, Michael Barfoot, 'Priestley, Reid's circle and the third organon of human reasoning', in R. G. W. Anderson and Christopher Lawrence (editors), *Science, medicine and dissent: Joseph Priestley (1733–1804)*, London, Wellcome Trust/Science Museum, 1988, pp. 81–9.

[47] For a discussion, see M. Barfoot, 'James Gregory (1753–1821) and Scottish scientific metaphysics, 1750–1800', Ph.D diss., University of Edinburgh, 1983, ch. 5, 'Knowing the nervous system: conceptions of nervous aetiology in the writings of Whytt, Cullen and Gregory', pp. 197–263.

[48] Jones, *Inquiry*, op. cit., note 22 above, p. 65. Jones saw the physician's application of laws of nature to effect a cure as analogous to the role of the legislator's, framing laws of society for the benefit of members. Dereliction of duty in the former was, in its way, no less serious than in the latter (p. 34).

[49] This was such an accepted feature of medical practice in Edinburgh that few writers commented on it explicitly. But see [William Graeme], *An essay for reforming the modern way of practicing in Edinburgh, wherein it is proved that the foreign method of paying physicians with small fees at a time would be of great benefit to the nation, if it were followed in Edinburgh, and the other Royal Burghs of Scotland, and do no hurt to physicians themselves*, Edinburgh, James Davidson and others, 1727, p. 13; and James Gregory, *Memorial to the Managers of the Royal Infirmary*, Edinburgh, Murray and Cochrane, 1800, p. 186.

enough to prove the soundness of a physician as a practitioner. Several of the professorial colleagues of these men would have been in considerably reduced circumstances, had it not been for a regular income from student fees.

It would therefore have been enormously difficult for Brown to acquire practice, even if he were impeccably orthodox in his views. As a medical radical and an extramural teacher his own prospects were bleak. The opportunities for those of his followers who had taken degrees, and remained in Edinburgh to practise, must have been virtually non-existent. This placed an apologist for the practical success of Brunonianism in a difficult position. Jones overcame this in part by recounting how Brown and his disciples had been consulted in private cases where orthodox medicine had failed. Some of these involved sick students; other cures were performed upon townsmen whose families would have been known to the local readership of Jones's book. There were also further details about Brown's management of his own gout to be drawn upon. However, this was at best a pastiche of *ad hominem* evidence and hearsay, and it required something more substantial to corroborate the appropriateness of Brunonianism as a form of practice. Jones turned to the Royal Infirmary to supply this.[50] The limited opportunities for physicians to practise in Edinburgh made it one of the few semi-public places open to Brunonians. They used their right of access to mount an assault upon the orthodox, antiphlogistic practice of medicine associated with Infirmary, University, and College physicians.

The sick poor offered ample opportunities for a physician-professor, or an aspiring young Fellow of the Royal College of Physicians who wanted to enhance his credentials for private practice. The Infirmary was a public gazebo, where news of success and failure was propagated by a social intelligence system involving patients, students, and managers. University professors ran clinical wards and gave lectures on patients; attendance at the Infirmary and clinical lectures was increasingly recognized as a crucial component of medical education. Students copied down clinical reports from ward ledgers, and attended more extensive discussions of particular cases. It was a complex medical bureaucracy based upon the transcription of records. Although the Infirmary actually got students somewhere near the patient's bedside, the professor had complete authority and dictated all the particulars relevant to the case. A considerable number of clinical reports and lectures, painstakingly transcribed by students, have survived. But there is little if any evidence of independent diagnostic judgement in them—that is, until Robert Jones published details of several cases from James Gregory's clinical wards in the spring of 1781.[51]

The matriculation album confirms that Jones signed up for clinical lectures in the 1780–81 session. He witnessed Gregory's practice and copied down the details of treatment from the ward ledger.[52] However Jones copied them for a purpose quite

---

[50] On the Infirmary, see G. B. Risse, *Hospital life in Enlightenment Scotland: care and teaching in the Royal Infirmary of Edinburgh,* New York and Cambridge, Cambridge University Press, 1986. For an earlier treatment, see A. L. Turner, *Story of a great hospital: the Royal Infirmary of Edinburgh 1729–1929,* Edinburgh, Oliver and Boyd, 1937.

[51] Jones, *Inquiry,* op. cit., note 22 above, pp. 188–307: cases of Alexander Hall, James Young, Bernard Stewart, William Goodwin, Catharine Neish, Betty Miller, Richard Thomson, and Betty Jackson.

[52] For further details of the hospital record system, see Risse. op. cit., note 50 above, pp. 43–56; 296–302. The original ward ledger from which Jones took his information is no longer extant. However, see Library

different from that of the majority of his fellow students. He used the cases to attack Gregory's practice as representative of the eclectic, empiric procedures of antiphlogistic therapy. Jones claimed that he had chosen Gregory, not through personal vindictiveness, but because he was acknowledged as the best of those practitioners to whom the students had access. The details of Jones's criticisms are too complicated to relate in any detail, but the general themes are clear enough.

Jones used the first two cases to show that Gregory had failed to distinguish between local and idiopathic disease of the digestive system. He claimed that although Brunonianism was only concerned with universal disease, it had stricter criteria for identifying local complaints based on some form of organic lesion. To act on the body's excitability in cases of local disease was useless and this is precisely what Jones said Gregory had done in the first case. Gregory's want of judgement had "tormented a poor dying creature for a number of days and [he] gave himself a great deal of useless trouble."[53] The second of the two cases was a genuine case of idiopathic diarrhoea. Here Jones criticized Gregory for confounding stimulating and debilitating procedures in the application of what Jones called a "farrago of drugs and remedies".[54] From a Brunonian point of view, Gregory's case history was a false species of evidence from which it was impossible to understand the cause of disease. Gregory's practice was presented as a form of inconsistent and piecemeal empiricism, comparable to that of the "Prince of Quacks", James Graham. Jones then gave details of how to cure the case on Brunonian principles using the gradual application of such diffusable stimulants as opium, coupled to a diet containing red meat and alcohol. The other cases analysed involved fever, haemorrhage, and dropsy, and each exposed further assumptions and unjustifiable features of the antiphlogistic cure. The common principle behind the various Brunonian counter-indications was presented as an application of Newton's second rule of reasoning, which would ensure continuity in patient treatment. Similar effects always implied similar causes; therefore, in cases where debility was the clear effect, it was fruitless to apply remedies which caused further debility. Instead, stimulating causes should be applied to produce stimulating effects. In this manner, Brunonianism offered the young practitioner a way of cutting through the arcana of practice and side-stepping the authority of professorial experience.[55] Diagnostic procedures were clear and

---

of the Royal College of Physicians of Edinburgh MS, James Gregory 3, Clinical notes, Edinburgh, 1780–81. This is in an unknown student hand and includes details of the same cases, together with extracts from clinical lectures based on them. Although some details overlap enough to suggest a common source, these notes are much sketchier than Jones's own. Jones also criticized the recording system in the Infirmary, claiming there were many omissions and errors (*Inquiry*, op. cit., note 22 above, p. 216). Therefore he made his own cases as complete as possible. A comparison of general details, diagnoses and care outcomes contained in Jones, the other casebook, and the General Register of Patients, which has also survived, tends to support Jones's point, and reveals many of the difficulties surrounding their use as a historical source today.

[53] Jones, *Inquiry*, op. cit., note 22 above, p. 211.

[54] Ibid., p. 201.

[55] Gregory did not reply directly to the Brunonian attack on his practice, but see *Conspectus medicinae theoreticae; or a view of the theory of medicine* (1778–82), translated from the original Latin, new ed., Edinburgh, Maclachlan and others, 1844, pp. 264–6. In his discussion of stimulants and sedatives, which was first published a year after the *Inquiry*, Gregory disputed the role of causal maxims in medical reasoning, such as those advocated by Jones, and appealed instead to the role of experience.

relatively uncomplicated. Was a disease local or idiopathic? If the latter, was it asthenic or sthenic? If the former, was the debility direct or indirect? All disease forms were accommodated under these categories and this step was justified by appealing to Newton's third rule of reasoning. It is not surprising that the College of Physicians was as troubled as the clinical professors in the Infirmary by Brunonianism, which represented a direct assault upon the arcana of practice. It identified the damage done by an unwarranted reliance upon so-called specifics in the materia medica, and called for the whole subject to be reformed according to "the principles of philosophical analysis".[56] If Brunonian principles were adopted, it would result in the deracination of a whole range of florid and exotic remedies which hitherto had bloomed, largely undisturbed, in the carefully tended gardens of college and hospital pharmacopoeias. This approach, together with the insistence upon substituting fresh observation for authoritative experience, enhanced its appeal as a set of rules for the guidance of the independent young medical practitioner. In short, Brunonianism was the educated physician's version of William Buchan's *Domestic medicine*.[57]

As well as the detailed criticism of particular cases, the Brunonian assault on Infirmary practice also had a broader dimension. Jones hinted at this when he stated that "the lives of our fellow creatures [were] subjected, especially in hospitals and dispensaries, to the dogmatic canons of credulous graduates."[58] Jones also briefly mentioned the wider role that Brunonian diet and regimen had to play in the prevention and cure of disease among the labouring poor. Brunonian therapeutics emphasized that too much exercise, coupled with a vegetable diet, led to dyspepsia, diarrhoea, schirrhus, dropsy, and fever. He added:

> The diseases prevailing among the poor people, who are commonly starved, and oppressed with assiduous excessive labour, afford many instances of diseased state originating from this source of direct debility.[59]

This theme was developed more fully in a pamphlet, which appeared anonymously a year after the publication of the *Inquiry,* entitled *A letter to John Hope.*[60] Hope was one of the Ordinary Physicians at the Infirmary and also Professor of Botany. Along with Cullen, Gregory, Francis Home, and Andrew Duncan, he was publicly accused, tried, and convicted of practising antiphlogistic medicine. Jones's *Inquiry* was praised several times in the *Letter,* where so many of his themes received a second airing as to

---

[56] Jones, *Inquiry,* op. cit., note 22 above, p. 59.

[57] See C. E. Rosenberg, 'Medical text and social context: explaining William Buchan's "Domestic medicine"', *Bull. Hist. Med.,* 1983, **57**: 22–42; C. J. Lawrence, 'William Buchan: medicine laid open', *Med. Hist.,* 1975, **19**: 20–35. For Jones's remarks on what he called "natural physic", see the *Inquiry,* op. cit., note 22 above, pp. 17–18.

[58] Ibid., p. 72. Jones made derogatory references to case histories published by Francis Home and Andrew Duncan. See Francis Home, *Medical facts and experiments,* London, A. Millar, 1759; *idem, Clinical experiments, histories, and dissections,* Edinburgh, William Creech, 1780; Andrew Duncan, *Medical cases selected from the records of the public dispensary at Edinburgh with remarks and observations; being the substance of lectures delivered during the years 1776–1777,* Edinburgh, Charles Elliot and J. Murray, 1778.

[59] Jones, *Inquiry,* op. cit., note 22 above, p. 126.

[60] *A letter to John Hope, Professor of Botany in the University of Edinburgh, and one of the attendant physicians of the Royal Infirmary; on the management of patients in that hospital; the contradictions adopted in Dr Cullen's 'First lines of physic'; and the superior merit and simplicity of the new system,* Edinburgh, 1782.

suggest that Jones was involved.[61] Just as Jones's book related medical reform to social issues of general concern, this pamphlet attempted to engage the wider population of Edinburgh on a specific matter.

Once more, institutional corruption was the theme. The argument throughout was that the sick poor suffered because of the stringent economy of the hospital, and that this was inconsistent with its status as a charitable institution. It referred to the widely known practice of friends and relatives bringing food which patients came to depend on for their survival. Hope's patients, in particular, were under-fed and over-bled. The diet schedules were reproduced and contrasted unfavourably with provisions at St George's Hospital.[62] It pointed out that most patients were already weak and what they wanted was food and drink, not a regimen which depleted them further:

> When a labourer has been hard wrought, ill-fed, and catches cold, you most absurdly suppose, that this poor creature is in a state of excessive vigour, and that his veins (forsooth!) are over full. *Quere*. Can transubstantiation be a greater absurdity? The miserable patient, however, is commonly bled, and purged, and blistered, and starved, and in short, reduced by every mode of inanition to a state of the most deplorable and desperate debility.[63]

By producing this pamphlet, the Brunonians made an important contribution to a continuing debate about the public health of the poor in Edinburgh. The proper care of the respectable sick poor in hospitals would be one solution to this problem; the Infirmary itself was dependent upon the whims of charitable virtue, and as as result, it lurched from one financial crisis to another. A less publicized but significantly larger institution, related to the same concern, was the Charity Workhouse.[64] Despite some municipal funding, it also experienced severe financial difficulties which began even before it actually opened in the early 1740s. In 1749, the Town Council applied to Parliament for a stent to be levied on the local population for the upkeep of the poor. This was successfully resisted by a committee organized by the professional and well-to-do sections of the community.[65] The parish heritors, merchants, guildsmen, and burgesses felt they had paid out more than their share. The Workhouse got deeper in debt and had to take out several loans. Voluntary contributions continued to be collected from parishioners. As a result, there was a resurgence of resentment against the Edinburgh poor provision, which coincided almost exactly with the appearance of the Brunonian pamphlet. In the same year, a time of famine and great scarcity of provisions in Scotland, John M'Farlan, a

---

[61] See ibid., p. 26, for a reference to Jones's exposure of Gregory's cases, with the prediction that it had "put a final period to the publication of *medical cases* from the *Cullenian* quarter."

[62] Ibid., pp. 8–12.

[63] Ibid., p. 27.

[64] For the general background, see R. A. Cage, *The Scottish poor law 1745–1845*, Edinburgh, Scottish Academic Press, 1981. For details, see City of Edinburgh District Council Archive, bay C, shelf 14, Minutes of the Charity Workhouse.

[65] For an account of the episode, see Jos. Williams, *Memorial for the Magistrates and Council of the City of Edinburgh, containing a short account of the Charity Work House, the reasons for applying to the legislature, in order to procure the establishment of a certain and equal fund for the maintenance and employment of the poor belonging to this City and Royalty, with answers to the objections against applying to Parliament for a poor rate, c. 1750.*

minister at the Canongate Church, published his *Inquiries concerning the poor.*[66] He opposed workhouses and claimed they were expensive because the poor in them were too well provided for. His view was refuted in 1783 by a merchant and treasurer of the Orphan Hospital, Mr T. Tod, who clearly felt that the burden of the poor had fallen inequitably upon the charitable shoulders of his sector of society.[67] Tod exposed what he saw as M'Farlan's Mandevillian arguments for reducing the provision for the poor. He felt it was a convenient rationalization for members of the professional and gentry classes, who were already reluctant to make voluntary contributions.

Clearly, the Brunonians wanted to mobilize the simmering resentment among the townsmen, and perhaps even win the surgeons and apothecaries over to their practices. They endorsed the widely held view that affluent and professional groups did not care about the unrespectable poor. What they added to the debate was a claim that this lack of charity extended to the mismanagement of the respectable sick poor in the Infirmary. However, Brunonian hopes for reform were over-optimistic. Tod did seem an ally when he attacked M'Farlan's socially-divisive and élitist attitude to the poor. But most of his book was actually devoted to defending the Edinburgh workhouses, on the grounds that they were much more frugally managed than their English counterparts. So the Brunonian message for public health went unheard. It was shouted down by a debate which turned not on the question of whether the Edinburgh poor should be fed as well as the English apparently were, but, in fact, on whether they were being fed and looked after as badly as they should be.

CONCLUSIONS

Jones's *Inquiry* helps us to reconstruct the content of early Brunonian ideology as it emerged in late eighteenth-century Edinburgh. This had three main dimensions. It involved a republican attitude to medical free-thinking, which related developments in medicine to the history of human understanding within political society. It stressed the role of induction as a reforming scientific method; and the application of Newton's rules of reasoning it favoured led to a distinctive account of life in terms of the excitability of animal (and vegetable) matter. Finally, it advocated a plan of cure based largely upon the use of stimulant remedies, which was perceived to have important consequences for the public health of the poor. Throughout, the intellectual aspects of reforming medicine associated with Brunonianism were inseparable from a political assessment of the physician's role and responsibilities in society. It now remains to examine whether the movement successfully used this ideology to change the Edinburgh medical community.

It is impossible to substantiate Jones's and other committed versions of particular episodes in the reception of Brunonianism. However, in one important respect, his account was probably very accurate. His attack focused upon members of the University, Infirmary, and College. From Jones's perspective, they were the conservative "Junto" of physicians who had collaborated to exile Brown, and to extinguish the enthusiasm which the Brunonian movement had initially generated.

---

[66] John M'Farlan, *Inquiries concerning the poor*, Edinburgh, T. Longman and J. Dickson, 1782.

[67] T. Tod, *Observations on Dr. M'Farlan's Inquiries concerning the state of the poor*, Edinburgh, James Donaldson, 1783.

Irrespective of Jones's commitment to the new doctrine, his identification of the sources of power controlled by Edinburgh physicians is a very plausible one. Given this interlocking élite and the institutional vantage points from which it opposed Brunonianism, it should not be surprising that no major structural changes occurred in the Edinburgh medical school as a result of the movement. The University and the Infirmary were never seriously troubled by Brunonians, and no apparent diminution of their appeal to medical students can be detected. However, the movement's failure to change such inherently conservative bodies would be an unduly myopic criterion for dismissing the historical significance of Brunonianism as a local medical, social, and political force. Brunonianism did not appear wholly by chance. Instead, it absorbed and reflected back wider changes taking place in Edinburgh society.

The height of the movement, during the late 1770s and early 1780s, coincided with a significant point in the wider political management of Edinburgh society.[68] Until then, local government had functioned effectively, with Edinburgh at the centre of a network of patronage which spread throughout Scotland. Administrations came and went, and even the coronation of George III did little to disrupt the structure and principles of the Scottish political establishment. Its stability and conservatism underlay the early success of the medical school. The University expanded rapidly from the early 1750s, and continued to grow throughout the 1770s. Its patron, the Town Council, helped the medical school by appointing able professors who continued to attract students. Physician professors increased their status and acquired more power and influence over the community. Although it controlled most general practice within the Town, the Incorporation of Surgeons was, politically, out-manoeuvred and disorganized.[69] However, things were to change quite rapidly.

The halcyon days of Argyll and Bute and their management teams ended, and, prior to 1785 at least, the new despotism of Henry Dundas was not yet fully institutionalized. It was a period of transition; and the hitherto quiescent and loyal capital of North Britain experienced an unprecedented period of political and social instability. Coalitions involving Rockingham and Foxite Whigs in central government gave more radical Whigs a higher public profile in Edinburgh. There were heated exchanges about the need for electoral reform in the local newspaper press.[70] The focus of this kind of Whig sentiment was the Erskine family. In 1780, the

---

[68] On this subject generally, see A. Murdoch, *'The people above': politics and administration in mid-eighteenth-century Scotland,* Edinburgh, John Donald, 1983, especially pp. 124–31; *idem,* 'The importance of being Edinburgh: management and opposition in Edinburgh politics, 1746–1784', *Scot. Hist. R.,* 1983, **62**: 1–16; J. S. Shaw, *The management of Scottish society 1707–1764: power, nobles, lawyers, Edinburgh agents and English influences,* Edinburgh, John Donald, 1983; and the essays in J. Dwyer, R. A. Mason, and A. Murdoch (editors), *New perspectives on the politics and culture of early modern Scotland,* Edinburgh, John Donald, 1980.

[69] For further details, see R. M. Stott, 'The Incorporation of Surgeons and medical education and practice in Edinburgh 1696–1755', Ph.D. diss., University of Edinburgh, 1984.

[70] The *Edinburgh Evening Courant* and the *Caledonian Mercury* make fascinating reading during this period. Along with political squibs about electoral reform and church patronage, the columns were full of debate about M'Farlan's book and the state of the poor. Details were provided about the times and places of Brown's and other extramural lectures, including those of Dr James Graham, who visited Edinburgh in 1783. There were favourable reports about the Society of Antiquaries. Also included were a range of advertisements of recent medical books (including Jones's own), and about forthcoming plays on medical subjects. Finally, a series of articles reporting and satirizing debates in the Royal Medical Society appeared

Earl of Buchan founded the Society of the Antiquaries of Scotland, which obtained a Royal Charter in 1783.[71] His brother Henry Erskine was influential in the Faculty of Advocates and actually rose to become Lord Advocate. For a brief period, the constellation of opinions, values, and attitudes by which Whig and Tory sentiment was more clearly distinguished in nineteenth-century Edinburgh, was also present there in the late 1770s and early 1780s.[72] However, the reinstatement of Henry Dundas and the French Revolution wrecked any prospects of a Whig administration. In Edinburgh, Henry Erskine lost his job, and the Royal Society of Edinburgh was founded. The Society of Antiquaries could not compete with a rival which adapted itself to the climate of extreme conservatism which descended in the last decade of the century. Nevertheless, while it lasted, it was a period of political, social, and intellectual dissent, which the Brunonian movement did all it could to exploit.

To Brunonians and others, it seemed that genuine cultural and political changes were in the offing; and it was upon these hopes that they based their prospects for the reform of Edinburgh medical institutions. At one point, they appealed to "some great man whose benevolence is supported by power" to reform the Infirmary.[73] In the event, no one with the right credentials was prepared to back the Brunonian case for medical reform, and no major changes occurred as a direct result of Brunonian agitation. The Medical Society did receive a Royal Charter of incorporation in 1778, while the Edinburgh Public Dispensary was founded a little earlier.[74] Henry Erskine was involved in both episodes, but it was Andrew Duncan, a more respectable Whig medical outsider with Erskine family connections, who obtained this patronage, and not the Brunonians. However, they were responsible for a degree of conflict and disorder in the closely related institutions which made up the Medical School.

Controversy spread from the Medical Society, to the University, and attended the Infirmary throughout the 1780s and early 1790s. Shortly after the publication of the *Letter to Hope*, the managers of the Infirmary attempted to restrict students' opportunities to walk the wards. The students retaliated by forming themselves into an association and made Beddoes their spokesman.[75] They succeeded in getting the managers to reverse their decision. Brunonians or crypto-Brunonians lay behind the

---

in the *Edinburgh Evening Post* during 1783. They were entitled 'Medical intelligence' and appeared in nos. 288, 290, 294, and 296. On 5 April 1783, the Society Minutes noted the decision to take legal advice on the matter. No proceedings were actually started, but the Society did tighten up its rules for guests attending debates.

[71] See S. Shapin, 'Property, patronage, and the politics of science: the founding of the Royal Society of Edinburgh', *Br. J. Hist. Sci.,* 1974, 7: 1–41. For the early history of the Society, see *Transactions of the Society of the Antiquaries of Scotland,* Edinburgh, William and Alex. Smellie for William Creech and T. Cadell, 1792, pp. iii–xiii; William Smellie, *Account of the institution and progress of the Society of the Antiquaries of Scotland,* Edinburgh, William Creech and Thomas Cadell, 1782.

[72] This analysis is adapted from D. Marshall, *Eighteenth-century England,* London, Longmans, 1962, pp. 480–521; H. W. Meikle, *Scotland and the French Revolution,* Glasgow, James Macklehose, 1912, pp. 1–40; and Dickinson, op. cit., note 39 above, pp. 195–231.

[73] Op. cit., note 60 above, p. 4.

[74] See Grey, op. cit., note 10 above, pp. 53–5; *A general view of the effects of the dispensary at Edinburgh during the first year of that charitable establishment,* Edinburgh, 1777.

[75] See *A narrative of some late injurious proceedings of the Managers of The Royal Infirmary against the students of medicine in The University of Edinburgh,* published by the students. The volume of Royal Infirmary Minutes dealing with the controversy has been "lost".

shadowy students' association, which was still alive and protesting when the student body was excluded from the ceremony of laying the foundation stone of the new college buildings in 1789.[76] Critical reviews of the medical syllabus appeared, and there was genuine concern over the illiberality of some professors who refused to allow references to Brown in MD theses.[77]

Inevitably, the clash with Cullenian ideas in the Royal Medical Society took on features of this wider struggle in the minds of those involved:

> We mimicked, or rather felt all the passions of an administration and opposition; and we debated the cure of a dysentery with as much factious violence as if our subject had been the rights of a people, or the fate of an empire.[78]

This process of perceiving the medical in terms of the political was even taken one step further by Jones, whose account of the perfections of republican government is also a plausible description of the Brunonian conception of health:

> So complete now was the whole system, so enlivened and invigorated through all its parts, that every principal member would act the part of the head, and every head return to that of a member. There was now, while all the parts of the community, supported, excited, and corrected every other, no longer any danger, either of despotism on the one hand, or of anarchy on the other.[79]

Brunonian ideology certainly developed themes which reflected both the wider political views of the nascent Edinburgh Whigs, and anticipated those of more radical groups in the 1790s. However, this does not necessarily imply that Brunonians were politically active in the pursuit of wider reforms outside medicine itself.[80] The evidence available suggests that their concerns were largely confined to medical institutions. There is one indication of some involvement outside this sphere, but it concerned local cultural politics, rather than wider issues of government. Thus, along

---

[76] Ibid., hand-written addition, Edinburgh University Library copy.

[77] See J. Johnson, *A guide for gentlemen studying medicine at the University of Edinburgh*, London, J. Robinson, 1792; and Francisco Solano Constancio, *An appeal to the gentlemen studying medicine at the University of Edinburgh*, 2nd ed., London, Mudie, Murray and Callow, 1797. The dispute about graduation theses involved John Wainman, and was specifically directed at Monro *secundus*, who refused to allow Wainman, among others, to cite Brown. See Beddoes, op. cit., note 16 above, pp. lxxxiii–lxxxiv; Jones, *Inquiry*, op. cit., note 22 above, pp. 369–75. Jones and others were particularly severe on what they saw as Monro's illiberality over this issue. This was because he was known to share the Brunonians' opposition to Cullen's doctrine of spasm. However, Monro sided with Cullen, Andrew Duncan, and other members of the establishment against them.

[78] See Mackintosh, op. cit., note 21 above, p. 25.

[79] Jones, *Inquiry*, op. cit., note 22 above, p. 158.

[80] It is remarkable how figures associated with the Royal Medical Society during the period were involved in wider political issues of one kind or another. Sir James Mackintosh has already been referred to. For Beddoes's various activities see D. Stansfield, *Thomas Beddoes MD 1760–1808: chemist, physician, democrat*, Dordrecht, D. Reidel, 1984. Maclean attacked patronage and nepotism in the Army Medical Department. John Allen became involved in the radicalism of the 1790s and left Edinburgh to join the Holland House circle. He became a noted constitutional historian and Whig political biographer. Thomas Addis Emmet, (mentioned in Grey, op. cit., note 10 above, p. 61), another political radical and President of the Society, was actually imprisoned for agitation on the Irish question. This led such critics as James Gregory to remark that the Society was more appropriate for the training of orators than physicians and surgeons: op. cit., note 49 above, pp. 207–15.

with Smellie and Stewart, Brown joined the Society of Antiquaries, and became its Latin Secretary.[81] Jones was probably typical of other Brunonians who identified with it as an expression of Scottish cultural independence:

> A society has lately been instituted in this place, which from the candid, judicious, and impartial conduct of its noble founder, in filling it with distinguished names at home and abroad, and cautiously fencing it in against the encroachments of those freezers of the freedom of thought, those suppressors of all improvement in every department of thought, those craftsmen, who impudently arrogate to themselves the exclusive right of converting all the arts and sciences into a machine of gain for themselves, will certainly do honour to the kingdom, if their intrigues could be kept out of it.[82]

As a movement, rather than just a set of ideas, Brunonianism was widely perceived to have made an impact upon medical culture in Edinburgh. During this period, the Medical Society began to encourage the experimental investigation of medical and physiological topics which had become controversial during the course of Brunonian debates there.[83] Looking back from the early years of the nineteenth century, a new generation of commentators felt that medical culture had changed. They claimed physicians had renounced the "factions" and "party" politics of systematic medicine, and had evolved into "a congress of eclectics aware of the imperfections of medical

[81] Brown's wider social and political connections are far from clear. On his relations with Smellie and Stewart, see Thomson, op. cit., note 11 above, p. 715. He also had strong Whig connections through Parr and Mackintosh. During this period, Brown founded the Lodge of the Roman Eagle, although Freemasonry was not associated with radicalism by such authors as John Robison until later. See J. B. Morrell, 'Professors Robison and Playfair and the "Theophobia gallica": natural philosophy, religion and politics in Edinburgh 1789–1815', *Notes and Records Roy. Soc. London,* 1971, **26**: 43–63. Despite strong connections with the Campbells, Brown is also reported to have been a sentimental Jacobite. Hence it may be more appropriate to think of him as adopting the social and intellectual symbols of dissent, rather than the aims of a particular political group as such.

[82] Jones, *Inquiry,* op. cit., note 22 above, p. 362. The National Library of Scotland's copy of Jones's book used for this essay has the holograph inscription "To the Museum of the Society of the Antiquaries of Scotland from the Author". Buchan was elected an honorary member of the Royal Medical Society and his letter of thanks was inserted in their minutes. It contained themes similar to those emphasized in the *Inquiry.* Buchan stated that if "properly directed", the Society would succeed in making medicine more scientific in the Baconian sense. He added: "The whimsical Arrangements of System can never but disgrace, deform and perplex everything that they mix with, [and] I am persuaded that the noblest of arts under your auspices will acquire fresh dignity [and] importance by being stripped of its *fantastic* ornaments." See Minutes, op. cit., note 35 above, 13 April 1782.

[83] See ibid., 3 January 1784. Once again, the minute book dealing with the period 1784–90 is missing, which might suggest that controversy over Brunonianism continued well beyond Brown's departure to London. Experimental research carried out on such topics as inflammation, irritability, and respiration during this period needs further examination to see whether they were informed by Brunonian themes. For example, Edmund Goodwyn performed a series of experiments on drowning in the Society during the 1780s. These were discussed in *The connexion of life with respiration; or an experimental inquiry into the effects of submersion, strangulation, and several kinds of noxious airs on living animals: with an account of the nature of the disease they produce; its distinction from death itself; and the most effectual means of cure,* London, T. Spilsbury, 1788. Goodwyn was briefly mentioned by Jones, as a friend of John Isaacson. Although Goodwyn did not mention Brown, his views were also discussed by John Franks, a London apothecary, who claimed they were consistent with the Brunonian view of life as a forced state. See John Franks, *Observations on animal life and apparent death from accidental suspension of the function of the lungs, with remarks on the Brunonian system of medicine,* London, H. Reynall, 1790, pp. xlix–l. Thomson's lectures on inflammation (op. cit., note 12 above) were based on experiments originally performed in the Society. Alexander Philips Wilson (op. cit., note 4 above, Appendices to vols. 3 and 4) also carried out experimental research on urinary dispositions in fevers, and on opium, there.

science".[84] Medicine was inspired by a more "liberal spirit" of inquiry than it had been in the last two decades of the previous century, and this had to be nourished if men hoped to discover the laws of scientific medicine. From this vantage point, Brunonianism, especially in the guise of its founder's works, was certainly perceived as a form of systematic medicine which expounded the philosophy of induction, rather than experimental research as such. Nevertheless, it was also credited with having set the methodological direction to the be followed by early nineteenth-century Edinburgh medicine as a whole.[85] In this sense, Brown appeared as a Janiform figure. He was frequently acknowledged as the first to advocate that medical truth should be sought scientifically in terms of laws of nature. Paradoxically, he was also the last of the eighteenth-century systematic prophets of the inductive method who failed to find it.

Brown also showed that the audience for medical knowledge was not always a captive of the University professoriate. The expansion of extramural medical education in late eighteenth- and early nineteenth-century Edinburgh probably owed as much to this aspect of Brunonianism as it did to the contents of the lectures themselves.[86] It indicated there was room in the Edinburgh educational market-place for competition from new ideas and approaches different to those associated with the University professoriate. If Brown could do it, young physicians and surgeons could also fill lecture rooms, and so pursue careers in a city where medical opportunities could be very limited. In this way, features of Brunonian ideology contributed to the general climate of intellectual freedom which emerged through the clash with orthodox University medicine. The movement laid the foundations of an anti-establishment counter-culture which spawned the Academy of Physics and other scientific societies.[87] Nor were extramural medical and scientific institutions the sole beneficiaries. Brunonianism made an early contribution to the Scottish tradition more usually associated with the founders of the *Edinburgh Review* and the early decades of the nineteenth century, when social and political events were more conducive to its further development.

[84] See *The Edinburgh medical and surgical journal: exhibiting a concise view of the latest and most important discoveries in medicine, surgery and pharmacy*, 1805, vol. 1, pp. 357–75. These remarks were made in the course of a review of William Cullen Brown's edition of his father's works. Once again, the credit given to Brown is balanced by a major attack on the principles of excitability. See also Maclean, *Practical illustrations*, op. cit., note 7 above, p. xl.

[85] See G. N. Cantor, 'Henry Brougham and the Scottish methodological tradition', *Stud. Hist. Philos. Sci.*, 1971–72, **2**: 69–89.

[86] A. Philips Wilson, John Allen, and even John Thomson all benefited from Brunonianism in this way, as did John Aitken, another prominent extramural lecturer based at the Royal College of Surgeons. He was a member of the Society of Antiquaries, and Grey (op. cit., note 10 above, p. 77) stated that Aitken proposed Buchan for membership of the Royal Medical Society. Elizabeth Cullen Brown (op. cit., note 16 above, fol. 1) mentioned her father's friendship with a John Aiken, as his name was sometimes spelled. Aitken's views on medical improvement, animal life, and medical method were very similar to features of Brunonian ideology. See his *Principles of anatomy and physiology*, 2 vols., London, J. Murray, 1786, vol. 2, p. 119; and his *Elements of the theory and practice of physic and surgery*, 2 vols., London, Charles Dilley, 1783, vol. 1, pp. v–vi; 5–7; 66–9; 77–9. For further details on him and other extramural lecturers around this period, see John Struthers, *Historical sketch of the Edinburgh anatomical school*, Edinburgh, Maclachlan and Stewart, 1867.

[87] G. N. Cantor, 'The Academy of Physics at Edinburgh 1797–1800', *Soc. Stud. Sci.*, 1975, **5**: 109–34.

Factors which affected the transmission of medical theory and practice, alluded to at the beginning of this essay, make it difficult to connect changes in Edinburgh medical practice to Brunonianism as such.[88] Unfortunately, there is a paucity of information about the activities of members of the Royal College of Surgeons with which to assess William Cullen Brown's claim that local practice was deeply affected by the stimulant regime. On the wider question of Brunonian influence upon British practice as a whole, matters are even less clear, and it remains difficult to escape the dichotomy of opinion at the time. In view of this situation, perhaps it is appropriate to give Mr Jennings the last word:

'. . . Towards sunset, as is usual in such cases, the delirium incidental to the fever came on. It lasted more or less through the night; and then intermitted, at that terrible time in the morning—from two o'clock to five—when the vital energies even of the healthiest of us are at their lowest. It is then that Death gathers in his human harvest most abundantly. It was then that Death and I fought over the bed, which should have the man who lay on it. I never hesitated in pursuing the treatment on which I had staked everything. When wine failed, I tried brandy. When the other stimulants lost their influence, I doubled the dose. After an interval of suspense,—the like of which I hope to God I shall never feel again—there came a day when the rapidity of the pulse slightly, but appreciably, diminished; and, better still, there came also a change in the beat—an unmistakeable change to steadiness and strength. *Then*, I knew that I had saved him; and then I own I broke down. I laid the poor fellow's wasted hand back on the bed, and burst out crying. An hysterical relief, Mr Blake—nothing more! Physiology says, and says truly, that some men are born with female constitutions—and I am one of them!'

[88] For example, there is some evidence of the adoption of more stimulant remedies in the Royal Infirmary itself. See G. B. Risse '"Typhus" fever in eighteenth-century hospitals: new approaches to medical treatment', *Bull. Hist. Med.*, 1985, **59**: 176–95; and *idem*, op. cit., note 50 above, which discusses the increased consumption of alcoholic beverages at the Infirmary around 1790. William Cullen Brown (op. cit., note 1 above, vol. 1, pp. ccviii–ccix) had no doubt these changes were more widespread in Edinburgh practice and that they were due to Brunonianism. For another viewpoint, see A. Philips Wilson, op. cit., note 4 above, vol. 1, pp. 679–84. Jones (*Inquiry*, op. cit., note 22 above, pp. 352–5, case of Thomas Collins) claimed that James Hamilton, one of the Ordinary Physicians at the Infirmary, had adopted Brunonian practices. For other viewpoints, see James Hamilton, *Observations on the utility and administration of purgative medicines in several diseases* (1805), Edinburgh, Bradfute, Bell and others, 1823, pp. i–xx; and Parr, op. cit., note 3 above, vol. 1, pp. 374–8, 650.

Medical History, Supplement No. 8, 1988, 46–62.

BRUNONIAN THERAPEUTICS:
NEW WINE IN OLD BOTTLES?

by

GUENTER B. RISSE*

INTRODUCTION

Since John Brown's system of medicine encouraged the therapeutic use of substantial amounts of opium and alcohol,[1] it later became, during less permissive times, a typical illustration of the dangers of addiction and dissipation. Brunonian treatment was held up as a prime example of medical ignorance in the age of agony, a tragic case of what happens when impaired physicians go mad. Several historians have echoed such indictments, one even claiming that Brown's mode of treatment "sacrificed more human beings than the French revolution and the wars of Napoleon combined".[2] Another looked at Napoleon's adversaries, quoting a report that more than thirty per cent of the wounded Austrian soldiers died in a state of inebriation, felled by Brunonianism and its massive doses of Rhine wine.[3] For Victorian sensibilities, the creator of these alcoholic cures had to be a coarse man of low habits, "morally deserving of the severest condemnation".[4]

Such criticisms fail to realize that the so-called Brunonian therapeutics were already practised well before John Brown decided to quit theology and devote himself to the study of medicine. For example, the 1769 edition of the *London practice of physick* described a type of medical treatment for certain debilitating types of fever termed "slow" or "nervous". Among the components of this regimen were beef tea, chicken broth, and light cordial liquors. In fact, during the height of the febrile delirium, the patient was to receive pure or diluted wine, the amounts to be administered determined by the level of the pulse rates which practitioners hoped to increase.[5] The same therapy was recommended in another contemporary publication, which strongly advocated the employment of alcoholic beverages rather than bleeding, purging, and vomiting.[6]

* Guenter B. Risse, MD, PhD, Professor and Chair, Dept. of the History of Health Sciences, School of Medicine, University of California, San Francisco, San Francisco, CA 94143-0726, USA.

[1] For an overview consult G.B. Risse, 'The Brownian system of medicine: its theoretical and practical implications', *Clio Medica*, 1970, **5**: 45–51.

[2] Johann H. Bass, *Outlines of the history of medicine and the medical profession*, trans. by H.E. Handerson, 2 vols. (1889), repr., Huntingdon NY, Krieger, 1970, vol. 2, p. 637.

[3] Heinrich Haeser, *Lehrbuch der Geschichte der Medicin und der epidemischen Krankheiten*, 3rd ed., 3 vols., Jena, Fischer, 1881, vol. 2, p. 762. The original anonymous report was *Regulativ zur bessern Heilung der Krankheiten ueberhaupt, besonders der Nervenfieber*, Heilbronn, 1796.

[4] Baas, op. cit., note 2 above, p. 635.

[5] *The London practice of physic*, London, W. Johnston, 1769, pp. 8–10. Such supportive therapy appeared virtually unchanged in the 1773 edition (pp. 9–13) and the 1779 edition (pp. 11–15). By 1797 the *London practice of physic* actually expanded this section but the treatment remained essentially the same (pp. 18–30).

[6] *The practice of the British and French hospitals*, 2nd ed., London, Baldwin, 1775, p. v.

Similarly, opium had occupied an important place in the therapeutic armamentarium since Sydenham's times. The English Hippocrates found it "so necessary an instrument in the hand of a skillful man, that medicine would be a cripple without it".[7] His use of the "liquid laudanum" as a painkiller, antispasmodic, and restorative did much to popularize its use. A companion of Sydenham, Thomas Dover, launched his famous diaphoretic powder for fever in 1732; its formula contained opium, ipecac, saltpetre, tartar, and licorice.[8]

For its part, the genesis of Brown's therapeutic ideas was inextricably linked to his personal experiences with gout. As is known, he suffered a severe attack of the disease in 1771 at the age of thirty-six. By his own admission, Brown consulted an unnamed leader in the profession—in all probability his mentor, employer, and professor, William Cullen—who diagnosed a gouty plethora.[9] Told to abstain from meat and alcohol, Brown allegedly went on a strict diet of porridge and vegetables and claimed to have drunk only water for the next twelve months. Whether he also received an opiate preparation for pain is probable, but went unrecorded. However, his apparent compliance with this regimen was not rewarded—in fact, Brown claimed to have suffered more painful bouts of the disease while following doctor's orders.[10]

Depressed, and increasingly sceptical about the treatment he was receiving, Brown conceived the idea that perhaps debility, not plethora, had been the cause of his gout. Perhaps Cullen's antiphlogistic regimen was the main reason for his further suffering. Eager to test this hypothesis so contrary to conventional clinical wisdom, Brown resumed his convivial drinking as well as hearty Scottish fare and was suprisingly rewarded with six years free from the symptoms of gout.

Unquestionably, Brown's personal experience with gout profoundly coloured his subsequent medical judgment. Because of his meagre clinical knowledge, the apparent "cure" planted in Brown's mind the seeds of scepticism regarding the soundness of such traditional antiphlogistic methods as strict diet, purging and bleeding, not to mention the veracity of its theoretical underpinnings. When the gouty attacks eventually resumed, Brown sought help in opium, especially the liquid laudanum or "wine of the Turks". His gradual addiction to the drug—he used and recommended single doses of 150 drops—only complicated his disabilities further and led him to mistrust the celebrated healing powers of nature, which he came to believe effective only for acute and self-limited ailments. "Perfect health in every aspect seldom happens to mortals", Brown admitted in his *Elements of medicine,* "only perfect acquaintance with the true nature of life can open the eyes of practitioners."[11] Instead of nature, physicians were called on to heal.

[7] Thomas Sydenham, 'Medical observations concerning the history and cure of acute diseases', in *The works of Thomas Sydenham, M.D.,* trans. by R.G. Latham, 2 vols., London, Sydenham Society, 1848, vol. 1, p. 173.

[8] For an overview see J.C. Kramer, 'Opium rampant: medical use, misuse and abuse in Britain and the West in the 17th and 18th centuries', *Br. J. Addic.,* 1979, **74**: 377–89.

[9] *The works of Dr. John Brown M.D. To which is prefixed a biographical account of the author, by W.C. Brown,* 3 vols., London, J. Johnson, 1804, vol. 2, pp. 114–15. This is the preface of Brown's English edition of the *Elementa medicinae.*

[10] A detailed account of Brown's illness is also available in Robert Jones, *An inquiry into the state of medicine on the principles of inductive philosophy,* Edinburgh, T. Longman and T. Cadell, 1781, pp. 106–27.

[11] Brown, op. cit., note 9 above, vol. 2, p. 55.

This more interventionist therapeutic stance was probably uncommon among contemporary British practitioners. Greater caution prevailed at the bedside. Credit and reputation could be more easily garnered by those healers who allowed nature to take its course. However, if physicians such as Brown rebelled against this passive approach because they believed that the human organism had a natural "tendency towards disease and death", then a more assertive role made sense. Indeed, Brown blasted all "alexipharmac" practitioners who primarily prescribed debilitating diets and evacuant remedies which, in his opinion, only exhausted the remaining vigour of patients such as himself, enfeebled by porridge and vegetables.[12]

Based on his personal experience and perhaps some selective clinical observations of others, Brown established the following therapeutic principles:

1. There is really no such thing as a healing power of nature purposefully acting within the human body; rather, the organism possesses a fair amount of natural energy or excitability capable of restoration to a healthy balance with the help of stimuli.[13] If there is an excess, the condition is called *sthenia*; the opposite deficiency Brown named *asthenia*.

2. Thus, there are really no specific cures for particular diseases or parts of the body. Every medical treatment affects the whole body through changes in the excitability, thereby correcting the sthenia or asthenia.

3. There is only one form of treatment: the administration of stimulants. In *sthenic* diseases one employs weak stimulants to reduce the excessive excitement—namely blood-letting, vomiting, purging, sweating, cold applications, low watery diets, reduced physical activity, and mental rest. Conversely, in *asthenic* diseases, one uses an array of strong stimulants to increase deficient excitement, beginning with a solid diet containing meat, wines or spirits, gentle exercise, fresh air, increased mental activity, and four stimulating drugs: opium, camphor, musk and ether.[14]

4. Although physicians have gradually classified remedies according to some particular pharmacological action, in truth they all act in the same way, namely as stimulants of the human organism. The choice of which remedy to employ should be entirely predicated on its inherent capacity and speed in accomplishing the therapeutic goal: stimulation. Thus, drugs can be distinguished as moderately or quickly diffusible depending on the rapidity of their stimulating action.[15]

5. It follows, then, that dosage is quite important for achieving the desired excitement, especially if this bodily quality can be measured in degrees, as Brown insisted it could. If the practitioner was uncertain as to the actual state of excitement, a therapeutic trial with moderately diffusible stimulants was recommended to detect the true level.[16]

Consequently, it is apparent that Brown's chief therapeutic rules, while shifting the emphasis of medical treatment from the traditional tempering of organic functions—notably in inflammation—to shoring them up via supportive measures, were clearly

[12] Ibid., vol. 1, pp. 49–54.
[13] Ibid., vol. 2, p. 206.
[14] Ibid., vol. 3, pp. 6–17.
[15] Ibid., vol. 3, p. 290.
[16] Ibid., vol. 3, pp. 292–5.

grounded in conventional forms of doctoring. His recourse to alcohol as both a stimulant and restorative broke no new ground. In fact, alcoholic beverages became widely available to all classes of British society, especially after the gin craze of the 1730s.[17] Brown himself was an active social drinker widely known in Edinburgh pubs where he fraternized with other students. Like many Scottish physicians, Brown used such establishments to see patients and make the contacts necessary to upward social mobility, especially membership in learned societies and perhaps a position at the local university.

Such a linkage between alcohol consumption, healing, and social acceptance is poignantly illustrated by an episode in Brown's life. Called to Inveraray in 1783 by members of the Campbell clan to attend their stricken leader, Brown arrived just in time to see the man dying. While announcing his inability to pull the patient from the throes of death, Brown, his daughter recalled, "dipped a quill in wine and water and moistened the [patient's] tongue [and he] at length was enabled to swallow wine." As on other occasions, "the Brownian doctrine in all the nicety of its gradual advances was put to the test by its illustrious founder. He remained at this house for about three weeks where he was idolized more as a demigod than man, and Major Campbell was eating and drinking his wine with his physician until Brown left him", presumably recovered.[18]

A matching testimonial for the effectiveness of opium—albeit on a member of the animal kingdom—comes from the same source. As Brown was dining at a friend's house in Edinburgh, the host brought a dying turkey into the room. "By my father's desire, fifteen drops of laudanum were poured down its throat", the daughter recalled, "the season must have been winter for there was a great fire and the *patient* was laid on the rug before it." The bird, groggy from the medication, slumbered through the evening, recovered, and "grew up one of the finest turkeys of the gentleman's rearing", another triumph of Brunonian therapeutics.[19]

I

Was Brown's approach to treatment really different from that of his contemporary colleagues? Perhaps the hospital practice at the Royal Infirmary of Edinburgh, as illustrated in numerous casebooks, can provide some answers.[20] In 1771, the year of Brown's first attack of gout, John Gregory, professor of medical theory at Edinburgh University, took care of a number of patients hospitalized in the Infirmary's teaching ward. Among them was a 20-year-old female suffering from "slow fever" who was placed on a supportive regimen, including "half a pint of red wine/day on account of

[17] For an overview, see R. Porter, 'The drinking man's disease: the pre-history of alcoholism in Georgian Britain', *Br. J. Addic.*, 1985, **80**: 385–96.
[18] 'Reminiscences of Dr. John Brown, founder of the Brunonian system of medicine, with a letter on the same subject, both addressed by his daughter, Elizabeth Cullen Brown to Thomas J. Pettigrew (1838)', National Library of Scotland MS 5173.
[19] Ibid.
[20] For more details, consult Guenter B. Risse, *Hospital life in Enlightenment Scotland: care and teaching at the Royal Infirmary of Edinburgh*, New York and Cambridge, Cambridge University Press, 1986, especially appendices A and B, pp. 296–339.

faintness", common beer, and panada.[21] Gregory followed the same approach in a smallpox case, a 48-year-old black servant who received generous doses of laudanum (25–40 drops) at bedtime and a routine of beef tea, port wine, and boiled barley.[22] Laudanum was also prescribed in patients with diarrhoeas, as well as intestinal cramps, for cough suppression, and even hysteria.

His colleague William Cullen, Brown's mentor, although less generous with alcohol, liberally prescribed beer—generally about a quart per day—in fever cases. His wine orders usually called for a daily pint of diluted wine (two parts water for every part of wine). In one instance, Cullen even went so far as prescribing a spoonful of diluted brandy "at two different times and repeated so that he takes double this quantity in day" for a 36-year-old male suffering from a fever and sore on his leg.[23] In fact, Cullen was quite aware of the dangers posed by an aggressive therapy in so-called "nervous" fevers which, most practitioners conceded, arose out of weakness. In such instances, wine was one of the popular stimulants recommended to overcome the constitutional debility.[24]

Like John Gregory, Cullen also employed opium preparations in a variety of ailments. As he explained to his students in 1772—perhaps Brown had sufficiently recovered from his gout to hear him—"opium with its narcotic quality is a stimulus that can be applied to the stomach for exciting vomiting, to the intestines for purging, to the kidneys as a diuretic, to the bronchia as a pectoral."[25] In spite of such a wide range of indications, a fierce debate continued about the nature of opium action. Did it impair nervous transmission? Was it ultimately a sedative with only a fleeting period of arousal? Questions remained about the actual potency and equivalency of available preparations. The issue of increasing "tolerance" to the drug—namely gradual addiction—did not perceptively engage the practitioners' concerns, perhaps because the existing opiates with their impurities were not as habit-forming as later refined products, notably morphine.

When, almost a decade later, Brown's disciple Robert Jones attempted to promote Brunonianism in Britain, he presented as number of clinical cases taken from the Edinburgh Infirmary to illustrate the deficiencies of the contemporary approach to treatment. Among them was a 28-year-old male admitted to the hospital in April 1781 with a tentative diagnosis of "typhus" fever. The patient, already nauseated and febrile, had received an emetic the day before admission, and presented himself with frequent vomiting and diarrhoea. During the next six days, hospital practitioners instituted a supportive regimen with Peruvian bark and red wine but to no avail: the patient's condition steadily deteriorated and after progressive weakness and fits, he

[21] Case of Elizabeth Fraser, in John Gregory, Clinical Cases of the Royal Infirmary of Edinburgh, Edinburgh, 1771–1772, MSS Collection, Medical Archives, University of Edinburgh.

[22] Ibid., case of David Rutherford.

[23] Case of Andrew Gray, in William Cullen, Clinical cases and reports taken at the Royal Infirmary of Edinburgh, by Richard W. Hall, Edinburgh, 1773–1774, MSS Collection, National Library of Medicine, Bethesda, Maryland.

[24] For summary of alcohol consumption in the Infirmary, see Risse, 'Beer, wine and spirits', in op. cit., note 20 above, pp. 224–7. A general reference on the subject is S.E. Williams, 'The use of beverage alcohol as medicine, 1790–1860', *J. Stud. Alcohol*, 1980, **41**: 543–66.

[25] William Cullen, Clinical lectures, Edinburgh, 1772–1773, p. 79, MSS Collection, Royal College of Physicians, Edinburgh.

died.[26] As before, such treatments were designed to prop up the perceived weakness of this "typhus" patient—an approach on which physicians had already reached a consensus.[27] Although the procedures were essentially "Brunonian", Jones severely criticized the repeated use of emetics and purgatives which were "undoing by one remedy the effects of another prescribed at the same time".[28]

A careful analysis of the management of fevers at the teaching ward of Edinburgh Infirmary in the decades between 1770 and 1800 discloses some remarkable changes. In the 1770s the attending professors used purgatives and emetics in virtually one out of every four cases, but analgesics (including opiates) only twelve per cent of the time, and actual stimulants (tonics and alcohol) with fewer than one in ten patients. If one checks for the 1790s, however, emetics had gradually fallen out of favour—used in fewer than eight per cent of cases—while the use of purgatives remained at twenty-five per cent, and that of analgesics nearly doubled, to twenty per cent. Whether such shifts can be attributed to Brunonianism remains unclear.[29]

Jones, nevertheless, provided a case study from the Infirmary to confirm the changes that had occurred in that institution. The patient, a 25-year-old soldier, was seen by one of the attending physicians, James Hamilton, for a fever. After a somewhat stormy beginning, he gradually recovered and was discharged as week later as cured.[30] His clinical improvement coincided with the prescription of red wine and other spirits following an earlier administration of purgatives. Never at a loss for an explanation, Jones characterized the exemplary cure as "having introduced and seen carried into execution a complete revolution of the medical art in the chief nursery of its practical part in Scotland".[31] In truth, this regimen was identical to that prescribed by John Gregory a decade earlier in the same hospital.

Still, one can unquestionably detect some greater liberality in the use of wines and spirits during the 1780s and 1790s at the Edinburgh Infirmary. Francis Home, another professor, gave white wine as a diuretic and red wine mixed with water (one pint daily) in several fever cases. One typhus fever case managed to get 34 ounces of wine between physician's visits (either a 24- or 48-hour period).[32] James Gregory, for his part, showed a penchant for ordering alcohol, especially in the "typhus" fever variety. Six to eight ounces of red wine and two pints of white wine, beer *ad libitum,* and gin punch, usually reserved for patients suffering from amenorrhoea or generalized swelling, were common prescriptions.[33] Both, in turn, together with their

[26] Case of Bernard Steward, in Jones, op. cit., note 10 above, pp. 225–42.

[27] See G.B. Risse, 'Typhus fever in eighteenth-century hospitals: new approaches to medical treatment', *Bull. Hist. Med.,* 1985, **59**: 176–95.

[28] Jones, op. cit., note 10 above, p. 242.

[29] These data were obtained by checking all cases listed as "fever" in the student notebooks and closely examining the various prescriptions.

[30] Jones, op. cit., note 10 above, pp. 352–4.

[31] Ibid., p. 355.

[32] Case of David McDonald, in Francis Home, Clinical cases, copied by John T. Shaaf, Edinburgh, 1788–1789, MSS Collection, National Library of Medicine, Bethesda.

[33] See Risse, op. cit., note 27 above, and James Gregory, Clinical cases of Dr. Gregory in the Royal Infirmary of Edinburgh, taken by Nathan Thomas, Edinburgh, 1785–1786, MSS Collection, University of Edinburgh. Among Gregory's 20 cases who received gin punch, more than half were females with menstrual or circulatory problems.

colleagues Andrew Duncan, Thomas C. Hope, and Daniel Rutherford, increased their daily use of analgesics in the treatment of fevers, including the use of opium preparations (see table).

Table: TREATMENT OF INFECTIOUS DISEASES AT THE ROYAL INFIRMARY OF EDINBURGH (PERCENTAGE OF CASES)

Drugs	Practitioners					
	John Gregory *1771-2*	William Cullen *1772-3*	William Cullen *1773-4*	James Gregory *1780-1*	Francis Home *1780*	Averages
Anodynes	14·5	3·2	1·3	19·7	20·0	11·7
Purgatives	25·4	25·8	17·8	18·7	26·6	22·8
Emetics	30·9	19·3	31·5	15·5	26·6	24·7
Tonics	3·6	9·6	2·7	14·8	4·6	7·0

Drugs	Practitioners				
	Andrew Duncan *1795*	James Gregory *1795-6*	Thomas C. Hope *1796-7*	Daniel Rutherford *1799*	Averages
Anodynes	23·0	27·0	16·6	25·4	23·0
Purgatives	38·4	25·0	22·2	41·1	31·6
Emetics	7·6	10·4	11·1	1·9	7·7
Tonics	23·0	20·8	22·2	3·9	17·4

However, these near-Brunonian practices posed an increasing financial burden on the Edinburgh Infirmary. By 1790, the hospital managers acknowledged the greater in-house consumption of port wine, and practitioners in the institution were urged to restrain "the use of that article within proper bounds".[34] By 1792, the authorities established a system of monthly reporting on the use of wine and porter beer hoping to curb their prescription. A year later, wine orders issued by hospital physicians had to be rewritten daily or the house apothecary would stop providing such alcoholic beverages.[35]

At the bottom of such restrictions, of course, was the financial condition of the Infirmary, struggling to maintain its philanthropic services during the economic austerity of the Napoleonic war. However, an increasingly negative attitude toward the unbridled use of alcohol, so eloquently expressed by temperance advocates, also began to influence medical opinion. One famous London physician, John Lettsom, suspected that those patients demanding beer or wine at dispensaries were "at the brink of destruction".[36] Some practitioners hesitated to continue generous

[34] Royal Infirmary of Edinburgh, Minute Books, vol. 6, meeting of 5 July 1790, p. 56.

[35] The monthly reports were instituted on 3 December 1792. By 4 February 1793 the apothecary was empowered to countermand old wine prescriptions written by the house physicians.

[36] As quoted by William Sandford, *A few practical remarks on the medicinal effects of wine and spirits,* Worcester, J. Tymbs, 1799, pp. 85–6. Such demands for alcohol can also be seen in several case histories from Edinburgh. One of Cullen's patients, a soldier with an eye infection, was noted to "relish the wine very much". A subsequent progress note reads: "Very little complaints but from want of wine." Case of John Davis, in William Cullen, Clinical cases and reports taken at the Royal Infirmary of Edinburgh, from Dr. Cullen, by Richard W. Hall, Edinburgh, 1773–1774, MSS Collection, National Library of Medicine, Bethesda.

prescriptions of alcohol "for medical purposes", to the extent that some visitors smuggled such beverages into the Edinburgh Infirmary to sustain the patients' habit.[37]

Finally, with regard to diet in the management of patients, Brown vigorously argued for "solid animal food" in the form of beef broths or roasted meat.[38] This indication held true for all asthenic conditions, in which the individual was presumably debilitated. Again, following his personal experiences with gout, Brown criticized the "low", watery, vegetable diets traditional in the management of fevers, and thought to be especially appropriate during the early stages when most patients felt nauseated or at least not eager to ingest substantial amounts of food. However, the use of emetics and other evil-tasting medicines often only perpetuated such lack of appetite, and seriously disturbed the stomach and bowels. When recovery began, such iatrogenic complications frequently hampered the healing process and led to other problems.

Not surprisingly, Brown attacked the dietary practices of the Edinburgh Infirmary, branding the institution as "subservient to the purposes of hunger and starving". "The ordinary allowance of the house would hardly support the vital vigour of a kitten", he wrote indignantly in an open letter to John Hope, one of the hospital's attending physicians.[39] "Your broth", Brown charged, "is commonly much better qualified to operate as an emetic than to nourish the system."[40] Relatives of patients smuggled food into the house, even if they had to bribe the nurses. After publishing the "common fare" of the hospital, Brown challenged: "I defy the healthiest man in Edinburgh to preserve his health fourteen days on your beggarly pittance."[41]

Again, a careful check of the Infirmary's dietary indications reveals that such professors as John Gregory and William Cullen certainly ordered beef-tea or "household broths" for convalescent patients, but not until the 1780s can one observe an increase in full diets with meat dishes, primarily ordered by James Gregory for "typhus" fever cases.[42] There are indeed accounts that nurses brought supplies of raw "undressed" meat directly to the teaching ward and allowed ambulatory patients to roast it in the fireplaces before eating the meat with potatoes and turnips—a practice that would have certainly sustained a number of Brunonian kittens.[43] Of course, just as in the case of wine and beer, such generous diets were formidable budget busters, and, in times of mounting institutional deficits during the 1790s, impossible to sustain.

[37] This was one of Andrew Duncan's patients who had apparently suffered a stroke. Observed Duncan: "So much addicted was he to their use (spiritous liquours) that he could not live without them." Clinical reports and commentaries, Feb.–Apr. 1795, presented by Alexander Blackhall Morison, Edinburgh, 1795, MSS Collection, Royal College of Physicians, Edinburgh.

[38] Brown, op. cit., note 9 above, vol. 3, pp. 6–8.

[39] The letter was signed only "Veri Amicus" (friend of the truth) but can be ascribed to Brown or one of his closest adherents on the basis of style and content. *A letter to John Hope . . . of the Royal Infirmary; on the management of patients in that hospital . . .*, Edinburgh, 1782, p. 7.

[40] Ibid., p. 11.

[41] Ibid., p. 12.

[42] See Risse, 'Dietetics', in op. cit., note 20 above, pp. 220–4.

[43] Royal Infirmary of Edinburgh, *Report of a Committee on the State of the Hospital*, Edinburgh, 1818, p. 64.

In summary, then, the influence of Brunonian ideas on the Edinburgh practice of medicine as exemplified by the management of hospital patients in the teaching ward is far from clear-cut. Under the direction of leading university professors, such patients certainly received full diets, alcoholic beverages, and opiates, sometimes typically "Brunonian" even before Brown had a chance to expound his system. The aforementioned shifts to a greater emphasis in restorative approaches owes, perhaps, more to patient selection rather than a generalized reversal in therapeutic rationale. James Gregory seemed especially keen on treating a kind of debilitating fever he called "typhus" and to this admission preference we owe some of the changes in medical prescribing. To call them specifically "Brunonian" would probably stretch the truth.

II

Let us next look at clinical experiences in prominent teaching hospitals on the Continent to detect signs of Brunonian practices. The first one is the Ospedale di San Matteo, affiliated with the University of Pavia. After the curriculum reforms of 1773, medical education began to flourish there, especially under the directions of Samuel Tissot (1781–3) and Johann P. Frank (1785–95). After his father's departure for Vienna, Frank's son Joseph, an assistant physician at the hospital since 1794, was appointed professor of medical practice at the university.[44]

By this time Joseph Frank had become a strong supporter of John Brown's system of medicine.[45] To illustrate his new approach, he published a number of clinical case studies of selected patients who had been seen in the 21-bed teaching ward of the Ospedale di San Matteo during the first six months of 1795.[46] In contrast to Edinburgh, here Frank tried to implement a specifically "Brunonian" plan of treatment closely linked to Brown's two disease states: asthenia and sthenia.

"How could one distinguish clinically between them?" asked Frank. Unlike his Edinburgh colleagues, who continued to express clinical differences within traditional nosological entities, Frank wanted to accept Brown's entire system of medicine and consequently follow its major theoretical premises. One logical approach was to take a careful history from the patient, not just ferret out key symptoms or previous ailments. The anamnesis was specifically designed to yield—à la Brown—an inventory of past stimuli which had affected the patient. Life-style, diet, home environment, perhaps polluted air, and psychological stress related to job or family

[44] Details can be found in G.B. Risse, 'Clinical instruction in hospitals: the Boerhaavian tradition in Leyden, Edinburgh, Vienna, and Pavia', *Clio Medica* (in press). See also L. Belloni, 'Italian medical education after 1600', in C.D. O'Malley (editor), *The history of medical education,* Berkeley, University of California Press, 1970, pp. 105–19.

[45] For details see Guenter B. Risse, 'The history of John Brown's medical system in Germany during the years 1790–1806', PhD diss., University of Chicago, 1971, especially pp. 199–210. See also Ramunas A. Kondratas, 'Joseph Frank (1771–1842) and the development of clinical medicine: a study of the transformation of medical thought and practice at the end of the 18th and beginning of the 19th centuries', PhD diss., Harvard University, 1977, especially chapter 5, pp. 201–15; and Kondratas's essay in this volume.

[46] *Ratio instituti clinici Ticinensis a mense Januario usque ad finem Junii 1795,* with a preface by J.P. Frank, Vienna, Camesina, 1797. In the same year appeared a German translation: *Heilart in der klinischen Lehranstalt zu Pavia,* trans. F. Schaeffer, Vienna, Camesina, 1797.

relationships: all were possible factors, potent stimuli which could, perhaps, be ascertained through a barrage of leading questions. Frank's goal was to determine the patient's diathesis or disease predisposition before becoming ill. Environmental factors, in turn, could be ascertained through careful weather charts available for Pavia and its environs, supplemented by data concerning current air temperature, barometric pressure, humidity, wind velocity, and rainfall.[47]

One of Frank's clinical cases typically illustrates his new Brunonian approach. The patient, a 22-year-old male, was admitted to the university hospital on 11 May 1795 with complaints of generalized body swelling. Through careful questioning, Frank discovered that two months earlier the man had had an episode of nausea and vomiting, with pain over the left side of his abdomen. This had occurred during the pre-Lenten *carnevale,* which the patient celebrated by drinking copious amounts of wine and eating salted meat. For the next three weeks, the man had felt feverish on occasion and, after consulting a surgeon, had a phlebotomy. At that point swelling had begun in the face, abdomen, and legs, a condition diagnosed as dropsy and unsuccessfully treated by conventional methods. Given the history of the disease and the failure of such traditional therapies as blood-letting and purging, Frank immediately made a diagnosis of direct asthenia and ordered a regimen of strong stimulants which included Peruvian bark, squill, wine, and a full diet. An abdominal paracentesis removed twenty-three pounds of water from the patient's belly. However, all measures failed to improve the condition and the man died ten days later. A greatly swollen pericardium containing purulent material was discovered at autopsy.[48]

While Frank considered the above case a pretty straightforward *asthenia,* too far advanced for Brunonian methods to reverse, other patients posed greater diagnostic challenges. For example, Frank admitted on 5 January 1795 a 19-year-old peasant girl from the nearby village of Trivolzio. She was breathing laboriously and coughing up some blood. Her problems were barely five days old and had begun with chills, fever, cough, and pain in the right side of the chest. Powders and wet cupping ordered by a private physician had not stemmed the complaints. Since her pulse was hard and fast, Frank hesitated. Both the gastrointestinal symptoms and pulse frequency suggested a Brownian asthenia, but the respiratory manifestations and pulse strength pointed towards a sthenic problem, especially a pneumonia.[49]

What to do in such a quandary? How could one find out? Frank followed Brown's suggestions of carrying out a therapeutic trial. Perhaps the disease was sthenic after all. The patient was immediately bled—ten ounces of blood were removed—then placed on a strict vegetable diet and given laxatives. Unfortunately, the patient's symptoms failed to improve and she became delirious because of her high fever. Then Frank announced that he had been deceived. The symptoms, after all, denoted a generalized weakness, complicated by the bleeding and purging prior to admission, not to say additional in-house measures which only aggravated the condition. A

[47] See Fritz Aicher, 'Der Einfluss der Brownschen Lehre auf die Therapie, untersucht an der von Frank in Krankenhaus zu Pavia behandelten Krankheiten', diss., University of Munich, 1933.

[48] Case of Joseph Biroli, in Frank, *Heilart,* op. cit., note 46 above, pp. 336–41.

[49] Case of Josepha Baruffi, in ibid., pp. 192–7.

strengthening, stimulating regimen which included Peruvian bark, seneca root, meat soups, warm tea, and Malaga wine was immediately instituted. A bedtime narcotic draught containing opium was designed to check the restlessness and promote sleep. Within three weeks, this patient recovered fully, leading Frank to re-emphasize the dangerous effects of purging and bleeding which wasted vital forces necessary for achieving a cure.[50]

Similar cases abound in Frank's hospital practice. In retrospect, it seems clear that his attempt to make Brunonian therapy workable at the bedside faced considerable odds but that he managed to achieve a certain number of successes. Frank's first and foremost problem was diagnostic uncertainty: asthenia or sthenia, that was the question. He used a number of "careful" trials to ascertain the nature of certain ailments, showing the same bias as Brown toward asthenic predispositions and conditions.[51]

Once embarked on a course of so-called stimulating drugs, Frank pondered their choice and above all, proper dosage. All his patients received some form of opium during their stay at the hospital, often as a bedtime drink, but also in the form of enemas containing laudanum or by mouth, thirty to sixty drops, to achieve higher "degrees" of excitability.[52] At the same time Frank was surprised to find that many of his patients claimed to have seldom drunk wine before coming to the hospital, an oddity in such a wine-loving country. He was fond of prescribing such heavy wines as malaga—less frequently white or red wines, of which he ordered between half and one full quart daily. Up to four quarts could be consumed in the form of diluted "wine soups". Like other would-be Brunonian practitioners, Frank realized that wine therapy was expensive and a great burden on the hospital's budget. Thus, he invented his famous *potus excitans* (exciting drink) composed of one part of distilled alcohol to two of water and one part honey. Other liquids were also employed to mix the expensive wine with sugar, eggs and nutmeg.[53]

A careful reading of Frank's work and an analysis of clinical cases at the Ospedale di San Matteo in Pavia inescapably leads to the conclusion that, like other so-called Brunonians, he treated his patients empirically although he repeatedly tried to justify his actions with reference to the Brunonian system. Like his father before him, Frank had moved away from indiscriminate purging and bleeding as well as the prescription of starvation diets in fevers. Brunonianism provided him with a welcome rationale with which to justify a supportive and strengthening regime more compatible with his own observations. Indeed, Frank considered the patient's clinical improvement sufficient proof that his regimen was correct, eschewing Brown's mathematical

[50] Ibid., pp. 196-7.

[51] For a discussion of Frank's ideas, see Joseph Frank, *Erläuterungen der Brownischen Arzneilehre*, Heilbronn, Class, 1797, especially pp. 96-8.

[52] Ibid., pp. 132-3. Unlike Brown, Frank advised extreme caution in the administration of opium, always pleading for small doses.

[53] A catalogue of the drugs employed by Frank at Pavia can be found in Verena Jantz, 'Pharmacologia Browniana, Pharmakotherapeutische Praxis des Brownianismus aufgezeigt und interpretiert an den Modellen von A.F. Marcus in Bamberg und J. Frank in Wien', diss., Philipps-Universität, Marburg, 1974, pp. 158-214. Her discussion of the *potus excitans* is contained on p. 185. Although restricted to Germany, this is a most valuable work on the history of Brunonian drug use.

calculations of the excitability.[54] His flexible interpretation of Brown's main principles brought Frank's therapy closer to the practices of many other European clinicians.

At exactly the same time, Brunonian therapeutics were subjected to similar trials at the bedside in Germany. These occurred in Bamberg, where the enlightened ruler of the Würzburg-Bamberg bishopric, Franz Ludwig von Erthal, had erected a new hospital.[55] The 120-bed institution opened its doors on 11 November 1787 as part of a comprehensive health care system for about 6,000 people, including 3,000 indigents as well as numerous servants and artisans, living in the vicinity. Linked to the university and its medical school, the Bamberg Hospital quickly became an exemplary training ground for medical students and surgeons. In fact, for the duration of Franz Ludwig's life, his personal physician Adalbert Marcus was able to persuade him to divert significant funds towards the operations of the hospital, making it a showcase and example to be imitated in other German lands.

With Marcus, a Göttingen graduate and highly respected practitioner, at the helm, the Bamberg Hospital established nearly ideal conditions for the care of its patients. There were nurses aplenty, one for every seven or eight patients. The institutional diet was varied and rich, eventually attracting middle-class patients to the ward. Most importantly, Marcus had *carte blanche* to order any expensive drugs required by Brunonian therapeutics. Indeed, the hospital pharmacist was so accommodating to Marcus' wishes that he went to great lengths in trying to minimize, through compounding, such unpleasant aspects of eighteenth-century drug therapy as the obnoxious odour of asafoetida, or the bitter tastes of Peruvian bark decoctions and opium powder preparations.[56]

Marcus was thoroughly acquainted with the new ideas of neuropathology expressed by Haller, Cullen, and Brown, and was anxious to test their application at the bedside. As he declared, this was one of the crucial times in medical history when clinical trials and bedside observations were necessary and useful. "At a time when the Brunonian system is ready to accomplish a total revolution in medicine, its clinical confirmation or reputation may save the lives of thousands of patients", Marcus announced, concluding that "the task of proving the Brunonian principles is the duty of all physicians".[57]

Although the Bamberg Hospital provided an ideal setting for Marcus' clinical experiments, like Frank he had to contend with the diagnostic difficulties surrounding Brown's two conditions: asthenia and sthenia. Without diagnosis, the practical application of Brunonian theoretical principles could not occur. Not suprisingly, emphasis was again placed on the clinical history as the most effective vehicle to establish an inventory of the patient's past stimuli. Perhaps even more than Frank, Marcus paid great attention to environmental factors and he collected extensive data

[54] Frank, op. cit., note 51 above, p. 134.

[55] For a history of this hospital consult Christian Pfeufer, *Geschichte des allgemeinen Krankenhauses zu Bamberg,* Bamberg, Kunz, 1825.

[56] Adalbert F. Marcus, *Kurze Beschreibung des allgemeinen Krankenhauses zu Bamberg,* Weimar, Industrie Comptoir, 1797.

[57] Adalbert F. Marcus, *Prüfung des Brownschen Systems der Heilkunde durch Erfahrungen am Krankenbette,* vol. 1, Weimar, Industrie Comptoir, 1797, p. iv.

about Bamberg's geography and climate.[58] As Brown had before him, Marcus believed that the cold temperatures of the winter months provided insufficient stimuli and tended therefore to cause asthenic diseases.

In 1797, Marcus began publishing a selection of clinical cases seen at the Bamberg Hospital and treated according to Brunonian principles. His findings seemingly confirmed Brown's own impression that, as a category, asthenic-type diseases constituted the overwhelming majority of sicknesses observed in medical practice. For the quarter April-June 1798, for example, Marcus admitted 136 patients to the hospital. Of these, 112 (eighty per cent) were found to have *asthenia,* 12 *sthenia,* and 12 local diseases. Of the so-called asthenic conditions, nearly half were labelled "nervous fevers" or "typhus"; among the others were cases of intermittent fevers termed "tertians" and "quartans".[59]

An analysis of some clinical cases as reported by Marcus himself is quite revealing. One 17-year-old male, a carpenter's apprentice, was admitted to the hospital on 25 March 1797 with chills and heat, stabbing chest pains, and great thirst. On admission, the patient had a high fever, difficult respiration, and a soft, fast pulse. Marcus immediately suspected an asthenic condition since the young man worked very hard and lived frugally in a drafty attic. Besides, there was a virtual epidemic of nervous fevers going around Bamberg. Based on that assumption, Marcus prescribed a stimulating regimen of Peruvian bark and Virginia root decoctions, supplemented with meat broth and wine. Unfortunately, the patient failed to improve, complaining instead of more chest pain; his face was flushed and the pulse fuller and stronger.[60]

At this point, Marcus quickly changed his mind about the diagnosis, now calling it a sthenic disease and blaming the shift to a recent change in the local weather with warmer temperatures, a westerly wind, and rising barometer. Cold fomentations were immediately applied to the patient, two four-ounce venesections ordered at one-hour intervals, a blister placed on the left side of his chest, and the drinking of cold water recommended. The temperature in the ward could not be lowered because other hospitalized patients suffered from asthenia and required a warmer environment. After several additional bleedings, the apprentice recovered and was discharged in two weeks. Marcus commented that although his management seemed to mirror the traditional antiphlogistic approach, he was still treating the whole organism in Brunonian fashion through a carefully tailored withdrawal of strong stimuli. Moreover, he conceded that even experienced physicians could be fooled by the patient's complaints and symptoms. Brunonianism in fact helped practitioners to focus attention on the potentially deceptive nature of symptoms and physical signs.

[58] This so-called "medicine of the environment" has been the focus of a recent review. See James C. Riley, *The eighteenth-century campaign to avoid disease,* New York, St. Martin's Press, 1987. For a brief analysis see L. J. Jordanova, 'Earth science and environmental medicine: the synthesis of late Enlightenment', in L. J. Jordanova and R. Porter (editors), *Images of the earth: essays in the history of the environmental sciences,* Chalfont St Giles, British Society for the History of Science, 1979.

[59] Marcus, op. cit., note 57 above, vol. 2, (1798). More statistics and a useful discussion are contained in N. Tsouyopoulos, 'Reformen am Bamberger Krankenhaus—Theorie und Praxis der Medizin um 1800', *Hist. Hospitalium,* 1976, **11**: 103–122.

[60] Case of Andreas Trunk, in Marcus, op. cit., note 57 above, vol. 1, (1797), pp. 91–101.

Old treatment routines, solely predicated on such external changes as responses of the body's healing powers, could be quite misleading.[61]

Another case illustrates Marcus' efforts to get away from what he perceived to be stereotyped responses to the appearance of symptoms, instead of a carefully-planned systematic therapy based on truly causal principles. On 15 January 1798, a 23-year-old cooper's apprentice from the city of Mainz came into the hospital displaying all signs of a fever. Again, Marcus confronted a hard-working young man frequently exposed to the wintry elements, and said to be suffering from a considerable amount of personal grief and trouble. Another asthenia? Indeed, the patient received a stimulating diet including meat broth and wine, together with liquid laudanum, and, strangely, cold water compresses to the forehead: the latter were usually part of a debilitating approach. Fortunately, the lad recovered within a week's time and Marcus was able again to sing the praises of Brunonian therapeutics.[62]

According to his multiple reports, Marcus seems to have had similar successes with a number of intermittent fevers, bronchial and throat ailments, and gastrointestinal troubles. His opium dosages never rose much above forty drops of liquid laudanum—a moderate dose—and this remedy was credited with saving the lives of individuals affected during Bamberg's dysentery epidemic of 1798. However, the cost of such stimulating therapies was correspondingly high. In 1798 alone, Marcus admitted, the Bamberg Hospital used 44 pounds of Peruvian bark and 470 pounds of pure alcohol. The numerous pharmaceutical preparations attest to Marcus' ingenuity in expanding upon Brown's four original stimulants, as well as his ability to prescribe without budgetary restraints.[63]

EPILOGUE

What then emerges from this analysis of Brunonian therapeutics? A well-known German contemporary, Franz Anton Mai, aptly summarized the advantages which Brown's concepts had brought to medical treatment. His remarks were anonymously published in 1798 as a pamphlet and widely circulated.[64] In the first place, Mai celebrated the Brunonian efforts to dismantle complex systems of disease classifications and avoid the usual pondering over what constituted precipitating or remote causes of disease. Next, he praised Brown's criticism of the tormenting methods of cupping, leeching, and blistering, as well as the endless prescriptions of emetics and purgatives which often only contributed to the patient's suffering. The fear that opium was a dangerous and sedative drug had finally given way to its more confident, and at times daring employment for the well-being of patients. Moreover, Mai explained, practitioners now seemed more aware

---

[61] Ibid., p. 101. This case finally listed as a "peripneumonia".

[62] Case of Georg Leidecker, in ibid., vol. 3, (1798), pp. 50–9.

[63] For details, see Jantz, op. cit., note 53 above, pp. 77–145.

[64] Mai's work was titled *Stolpertus, ein junger Artz am Krankenbette* and published anonymously as simply "from a patriotic inhabitant of the Palatinate". The first two pamphlets, dealing with pre-Brunonian practice, were published in Mannheim in 1777 and 1778 respectively.

of the complementary role which dietary factors played in their healing strategies, and they now also carefully checked drug dosages and their effects.[65]

Of course, no reforms could occur without some trade-offs. Mai was keenly aware of the pitfalls and serious shortcomings of Brunonian therapy. For a system to rely extensively on the patient's history could be dangerous. Patients often had no intention, or lacked the ability, to communicate their complaints in great detail. From those who would and could, a veritable flood of accounts of trivial and often imaginary symptoms could overwhelm the practitioner, then forced to select those which seemed significant for subsequent management. Social class differences between patient and healer created language barriers, misunderstanding, and suspicion.[66] There was always omissions of embarassing facts, even when the social impediments were non-existent. If the clinical history alone provided the decisive inventory of past stimulants, physicians would inevitably err.[67]

Assuming that such diagnostic difficulties could be mastered, and a clear plan of cure outlined, how could practitioners be successful? Given the unpredictable progress of the patient's sickness, Mai and others thought that Brunonianism could succeed only if close clinical supervision was maintained. This meant that the occasional visits to private patients and the routine ward rounds in the hospital were insufficient. As the choice of drugs and changes in dosages, closely tailored to the needs of individual patients, were crucial to the achievement of therapeutical effects, Brunonian practitioners needed to check their patients more often, in fact every three hours during critical stages of their illnesses.[68]

In sum, Brunonian therapeutics, in so far as one can speak of a supportive plan of treatment de-emphasizing the traditional antiphlogistic interventions, became a rallying point for practitioners aware of the unfavourable side effects of purging, vomiting, and bleeding. It gave such physicians a justification to break openly with established practices in selected clinical instances for which their previous experience clearly led them to anticipate iatrogenic effects from specific approaches. In Britain, as noted, shifts in treatment occurred without the need to label them particularly "Brunonian". In all instances, however, both the depleting and stimulating regimens were components of traditional eighteenth-century therapeutics.

For others, Brunonianism provided the temporary illusion that contemporary medical principles could indeed be applied at the bedside. Instead of forcing practitioners to simply trust their instincts, an approach widely disparaged as blind empiricism and equated with quackery, healing measures could be explained and defended as logical consequences of laws explaining health and disease. This was certainly true for the treatment accorded to individuals at Pavia and Bamberg. Both

[65] Franz A. Mai, *Stolpertus, ein junger Brownianer am Krankenbette,* Mannheim, Schwan u. Goetz, 1798, p. 8. For a good summary of Mai's medical career see Eduard Seidler, *Lebensplan und Gesundheitsführung: Franz Anton Mai und die medizinische Aufklärung in Mannheim,* Mannheim, Boerhringer, 1975.

[66] Ibid., pp. 20–9.

[67] "Stolpertus, please do not be fashionable and arrive at a rather hasty, authoritative diagnosis of asthenia or sthenia when confronted with a patient", Mai advised. Ibid., p. 31. The very name Stolpertus indicates "one who stumbles"—presumably at the bedside.

[68] Ibid., p. 87.

Joseph Frank and Adalbert Marcus were thoughtful physicians, eager to manage their patients according to rational therapeutic plans derived from Brown's chief postulates. To implement them, practitioners needed to acquire a more complete knowledge of their patients, including life-style, occupation, living conditions, diet, previous illnesses, and mental status, as part of a comprehensive inventory of previous stimuli which would help in distinguishing the Brunonian asthenia from sthenia.[69]

In the final analysis, however, Brunonian therapeutics in the sense of a strict application of Brown's theoretical principles was doomed from the start. The impossibility of consistently judging the degree of bodily excitability exhibited by individual patients created confusion. As the above examples illustrate, the criteria for a clinical distinction between states of asthenia and sthenia remained fuzzy. Since there was no compass to chart a consistent healing plan, physicians vacillated between depletion and stimulation just as they had done before Brunonianism. Purging could certainly be harmful to a number of conditions, and a supportive regimen beneficial to weakened patients.

Even if such experienced practitioners as the Franks and Marcus were temporarily convinced that they could make diagnostic distinctions based on Brown's principles, they then encountered a formidable hurdle in designing their cures: lack of understanding concerning the effects of the drugs they sought to administer. Brunonian therapeutics called for a wholesale reclassification of the existing materia medica as well as a better distinction between the effects of disease and the remedies administered to counter its manifestations. Indeed, adherents of Brown's system demanded a more scientific knowledge of drugs and the principles of pharmacological action in human beings.[70]

Finally, Brunonian therapeutics provided a brief moment of excitement for physicians who chafed at the shackles imposed on their treatments by the traditional belief in the healing forces of nature. Some of them were tired of simply being the man-servants of their patients' postulated ability eventually to overcome illness. Others became convinced that such a passive attitude led to many victories of disease over the sick. Professional caution and ignorance may have favoured the traditional expectant approach; but was it not time to seek actively an understanding of the bodily processes of disease, diagnose them, find their cause, and, armed with such insights, actually reverse them with the help of a carefully planned strategy of diet and drugs?[71]

Unfortunately, such knowledge was as yet unavailable, and the Brunonian effort, though boldly conceived and executed, failed. Looking at the balance in human lives affected by these treatments—as older historians have done—yields a mixed picture. Those individuals whose lives were saved because of less purging and bleeding can be matched with a perhaps equal number of others over-medicated with opium,

---

[69] Risse, op. cit., note 45 above, pp. 324–35.

[70] See, for example, Johann J. Loos, *Entwurf einer medizinischen Pharmacologie nach den Principien der Erregungstheorie*, Erlangen, Walker, 1802.

[71] For more details, G.B. Risse, 'Kant, Schelling, and the early search for a philosophical "science" of medicine in Germany', *J. Hist. Med.*, 1972, **27**: 145–58.

camphor, and alcohol, of whom some, like Brown himself, became addicted in the process. Thus, the promise of a total revolution in clinical medicine was not fulfilled.[72] Marcus' prospect of saving the lives of thousands of patients failed to materialize. In the end, even the Franks and Marcus abandoned Brunonianism.

However, every medical development has enduring effects. Besides the renewed emphasis on careful bedside observation, history-taking, diet, drug dosage, and perception of the effects which such foodstuffs and medications have on the human organism, Brunonian therapeutics achieved something of lasting importance: a popular awareness of our expendable energy levels and need to restore them with the help of hearty drink, food, and tonics. Here is the medical rationale for our cocktail hour or pub visit after a day of hard work!

[72] For a brief overview of the use of alcohol see M. Keller, 'Alcohol in health and disease: some historical perspectives', *Ann. NY Acad. Sci.,* 1966, **133**: 821–2. More detail is in, Chauncey D. Leake and Milton Silverman, *Alcoholic beverages in clinical medicine,* Chicago, Year Book Medical Publications, 1966. On nineteenth-century Britain see J.H. Warner, 'Physiological theory and therapeutic explanation in the 1860s: the British debate on the medical use of alcohol', *Bull. Hist. Med.,* 1980, **54**: 235–57.

Medical History, Supplement No. 8, 1988, 63–74.

THE INFLUENCE OF JOHN BROWN'S IDEAS IN GERMANY

by

NELLY TSOUYOPOULOS*

The German reception of John Brown's system of medicine was paradoxical. During Brown's lifetime (1735–1788), when his work was becoming well known in England and the other European countries, during all this time, there was not the least interest in his medical ideas in Germany. "It is remarkable", wrote Coleridge, "that in Germany, where every thing new in foreign Literature is so quickly noticed, Brown's Elements should have been published 12 years before they were once alluded to, a few cursory sentences in Baldinger's Magazine excepted".[1]

Ten years after the appearance of Brown's *Elementa medicinae,* in 1790, Dr Christoph Girtanner, a well-known physician in Göttingen, published a paper in a French journal based on Brown's work, without mentioning Brown at all.[2] When the plagiarism was discovered a year later, the incident was much discussed; but even this small scandal did not help to make Brown popular in Germany. The silence about him and his ideas continued until 1795, when a sudden interest in him arose and he was soon well known all over Germany and across the border into the other German-speaking countries, Austria and Switzerland. Before the end of the century John Brown was one of the most famous medical men in Germany.

The first place to see the advancement of Brunonianism was Bamberg, in southern Germany, where its main exponent was Andreas Röschlaub (1768–1835), a famous physician at the hospital and professor at the university.[3] In 1793, a friend who had been visiting Pavia gave Röschlaub, still a student, a copy of Brown's *Elementa medicinae.* Röschlaub was very enthusiastic about it and he sent it at once to Professor Adam M. Weikard (1742–1803) in Fulda, a former physician-in-ordinary to Catherine of Russia, who was considered to be a progressive physician. Röschlaub was not mistaken in his choice. Brown's work impressed Weikard, who in 1794 arranged the first German printing of the original text from the Italian edition.[4] A year later, in 1795, Weikard published his own translation of the *Elementa medicinae,* the first presentation of Brown's work in German.[5]

* Prof. Dr Nelly Tsouyopoulos, Westfälische Wilhelms-Universität, Institut für Theorie und Geschichte der Medizin, Waldeyerstrasse 27, 4400 Münster, Federal Republic of Germany.

[1] Kathleen Coburn (editor), *The notebooks of Samuel Taylor Coleridge,* London, Routledge & Kegan Paul, 1957, vol. 1, p. 389.

[2] *Journal de physique, de chimie et d'histoire naturelle . . . par M. l'Abbé Rozier* [Paris], 1790, **36:** pt. 1, p. 422, pt. 2, p. 139.

[3] Nelly Tsouyopoulos, *Andreas Röschlaub und die Romantische Medizin,* Medizin in Geschichte und Kultur, Bd. 14, Stuttgart and New York, Gustav Fischer, 1982.

[4] By Pietro Moscati, (1794).

[5] Adam Melchior Weikard, *Johann Browns' Grundsätze der Arzneilehre aus dem Lateinischen übersetzt,* Frankfurt, 1795; 2nd ed., 1798.

As early as 1796, a year after Weikard's translation, a second translation of the *Elementa,* by Christof Pfaff, appeared. A second edition of this translation, published in 1798, included a supplement with a critical review of Brown's ideas.[6]

Meanwhile, Röschlaub also made a translation, but, out of respect for Weikard, he did not publish this until Weikard's second edition went out of print. Röschlaub's translation, under the title *John Brown's sämtliche Werke,* appeared in 1806–7 in three volumes.[7] This was the last translation of Brown's work into German.

Röschlaub and Adalbert Marcus, the director of the famous hospital in Bamberg, together successfully worked out the Brunonian system of medicine, and as early as 1797 they published the results of their collaboration.[8] Departing from Brunonian ideas, they created a new system, the so-called *Erregbarkeitstheorie* (excitability theory). Röschlaub presented this system in his major work, the *Untersuchungen.* The first and second volumes, published in 1798, went out of print so quickly that a second edition followed before the third volume of the first edition could be published in 1800.[9] Röschlaub and Marcus transformed Bamberg into an excellent, and famous, intellectual and medical centre to which students came from as far as America.[10]

In 1799 Röschlaub began editing a journal, known as "Röschlaub's Magazine", which for the next ten years would be the main forum of Brunonian medicine.[11]

Of course there were also opponents to Brunonianism in Germany. In the beginning these could be found among conservative doctors, the so-called "eclectics", who believed that everything new was acceptable only if it could be reconciled with the principles of traditional medicine. The most prominent was Christoph W. Hufeland (1762–1836). As early as 1797, Hufeland began to defend traditional medicine against the revolutionary tendencies of Röschlaub and Brown.[12] A true ecletic, Hufeland was later more diplomatic towards the movement. During the years of its great success he visited Röschlaub and Marcus at the hospital in Bamberg and he tried, in later works, to show that Brunonianism and the excitability theory were compatible with traditional medicine.[13]

A radical opponent of Brunonianism and Röschlaub outside the medical profession was Hufeland's friend, the conservative author and politician August von Kotzebue,

[6] Christof Heinrich Pfaff, *John Brown: System der Heilkunde begleitet von einer neuen kritischen Abhandlung über die Brownschen Grundsätze,* Copenhagen, 1798; 3rd ed., 1804.

[7] Andreas Röschlaub (translator and editor), *John Brown's sämtliche Werke,* 3 vols., Frankfurt, 1806–7. Subsequent references to Brown's writings will use this edition.

[8] Adalbert F. Marcus, *Prüfung des Brownschen Systems der Heilkunde durch Erfahrungen am Krankenbette,* vol. 1, Weimar, Industrie Comptoir, 1797.

[9] Andreas Röschlaub, *Untersuchungen über Pathogenie oder Einleitung in die medizinische Theorie,* 3 vols., Frankfurt, 1798–1800; 2nd rev. ed., *Untersuchungen über Pathogenie oder Einleitung in die Heilkunde,* 3 vols., Frankfurt, 1800–3. Subsequent references will be to this edition.

[10] According to Röschlaub's contemporary biographer, Joachim Heinrich Jäck. See, 'Dr. A. Röschlaub', *Allgemeine medizinische Annalen des 19. Jahrhunderts* [Altenburg], 1814, pp. 702–14.

[11] *Magazin der Vervollkommnung der theoretischen und praktischen Heilkunde* [Frankfurt], 10 vols., 1799–1809.

[12] Primarily in articles published in his famous and very influential *Journal der praktischen Arzneikunde und Wundarzneikunst* [Jena], 1795–1844. For example, 'Bemerkungen über die Brownsche Praxis', in ibid., 1797, **12:** 12–150, 318–49.

[13] See, Hans Joachim Schwanitz, *Homöopathie und Brownianismus 1795–1844: zwei wissenschafts-theoretische Fallstudien aus der praktischen Medizin,* Medizin in Geschichte und Kultur Bd. 15, Stuttgart and New York, Gustav Fischer, 1983, pp. 70–2; Tsouyopoulos, op. cit., note 3 above, pp. 57, 154–6.

one of the most popular and influential personalities in Germany. His numerous plays dominated the stage. In several of his comedies Kotzebue attacked Brunonianism in a very polemical manner, and ridiculed the Brunonian doctors. The student Karl Ludwig Sand murdered Kotzebue, a major representative of reactionary politics and reactionary literary agitation, in 1819.[14]

In 1799 the renowned *Allgemeine Literatur Zeitung* published a long, critical article reviewing Brunonian literature in Germany to that date.[15] The same year, in Röschlaub's *Magazin*, there appeared a short reply to this criticism by the philosopher Schelling.[16] This publication marked the beginning of the second period of Brunonian influence in Germany.

Schelling had mentioned John Brown in the *Weltseele* (1798) but was rather critical towards his ideas.[17] Soon after, under the influence of Röschlaub, he changed his mind, a conversion obvious in *The first outline of a system of a philosophy of nature*, published at the end of 1799.[18] There began close and productive co-operation between Schelling and Röschlaub, culminating in Schelling's visit to Röschlaub in Bamberg and his lectures on *Naturphilosophie* at the university there in 1800.[19] This new combination of Brown and Röschlaub's excitability theory with Schelling's *Naturphilosophie* met an enthusiastic reception and was very influential not only at the German universities but also on practical medicine.

But this initial phase did not last very long. Röschlaub and Schelling began to have serious differences which led, in 1805, to their final estrangement. In 1805 Schelling founded a new journal, *Die Jahrbücher der Medizin als Wissenschaft*, edited by himself and Adalbert Marcus. In fact it was a gesture against Röschlaub's *Magazin*.[20] The quarrel divided the Brunonians into two partisan groups, each criticizing the other, which discredited the whole movement. Most of the physiologists, like Franz von Walther, Ignaz Döllinger and L. Oken, followed Schelling's *Naturphilosophie*; while the pathologists (E. Grossi, J. W. Ringseis, and J. L. Schönlein) preferred Röschlaub. But this distinction is relative. The physiologists in Schelling's train appeared to be more

---

[14] Gerhard Otto Hölzke, 'Die medizinischen Lehren John Browns und Franz Joseph Galls in der dichterischen Darstellung August von Kotzebues', diss., Friedrich-Schiller-Universität Jena, 1958; see also Werner Leibbrand, 'August von Kotzebue und die Ärzte', *Medizinische Welt* [Berlin], 1934, **8**: 282–4; and Fritjof Stock, *Kotzebue im literarischen Leben der Goethezeit*, Düsseldorf, Bertelsmann, 1971.

[15] The author was Dr Johann S. Stieglitz, a medical practitioner in Göttingen. 'Anzeige verschiedener Schriften das Brownsche System betreffend', *Allgemeine Literatur-Zeitung*, 1799, **48**: 377–82, 465–70.

[16] 'Einige Bemerkungen aus Gelegenheit einer Rezension Brownscher Schriften in der A.L.Z.', *Magazin*, op. cit., note 11 above, 1799a, **2**: 255–62.

[17] Friedrich Wilhelm Joseph Schelling, *Von der Weltseele. Eine Hypothese der höheren Physik zur Erklärung des allgemeinen Organismus* [1798], in *Sämmtliche Werke*, pt. I, vol. 2, Stuttgart and Augsburg, 1857, p. 505.

[18] *Erster Entwurf eines Systems der Naturphilosophie* [1799], in ibid., vol. 3 (1858). See also Nelly Tsouyopoulos, 'Schellings Konzeption der Medizin als Wissenschaft und die "Wissenschaftlichkeit" der modernen Medizin', in Ludwig Hasler (editor), *Schelling: seine Bedeutung für eine Philosophie der Natur und der Geschichte*, Referate und Kolloquien der internationalen Schelling-Tagung Zürich 1979, Stuttgart and Bad Cannstatt, Frommann-Holzboog, 1981, pp. 107–16.

[19] Tsouyopoulos, op. cit., note 3 above, p. 57.

[20] Ibid., pp. 162ff. See also Bernhard Krabbe, 'Die "Jahrbücher der Medizin als Wissenschaft" (1805–1808). Untersuchungen zu einer medizinisch-philosophischen Zeitschrift der Romantik mit unveröffentlichen Briefen aus Schellings Nachlass', diss., Westfälische Wilhelms-Universität, Münster, 1984.

successful than the pathologists.[21] Röschlaub was isolated and his *Magazin* ceased publication after 1809. Discussion of Brunonianism then became rare.

But soon thereafter a new wave of interest in John Brown became evident: arising about 1813, it culminated during the years 1815–20. In 1816 Röschlaub founded a new journal in which he published several articles, most of them about John Brown's method.[22] Hufeland, the main opponent of Brown and Röschlaub, began, after 1816, to open his *Journal* to the partisans of Brunonianism. Hufeland himself wrote several articles about John Brown, in 1819, 1822, and 1829, and compared Brown with Galen.

The reason for the renewal of interest in John Brown at this time was the success and popularity of the French physician Broussais, whose theory was also based on the doctrines of John Brown.[23]

The interest in, and discussion about, John Brown is very well documented in the medical literature of this period. During the years 1813–14 a severe typhus epidemic arose in Germany. All doctors and practitioners were engaged in the struggle against it and a considerable number of typhus studies appeared then or immediately after.[24]

Of course there were the usual quarrels between renowned physicians. One of the most prominent rivalries was between the old friends Marcus and Röschlaub. Marcus became an enthusiastic partisan of Broussais' inflammation theory; while Röschlaub defended the classical theory of Brown. The numerous treatises about epidemic typhus show that Brunonianism was still the central theme of discussion among medical professionals, and the point of departure for all serious considerations concerning practical medicine.

The year 1819 saw the beginning of political anti-liberalism which would influence all aspects of German life. Sand's murder of Kotzebue, on 23 March 1819, gave Metternich a welcome pretext to force new restrictive laws upon Germany. The so-called *Karlsbader Beschlüsse* were accepted by the *Bundestag* in Frankfurt and after 20 September 1819 they were established as Federal law. These resolutions were mainly targeted at the student's union, the independence of the universities, and the liberty of the press. Intellectual life was thus reduced to a minimum, liberal professors were persecuted, and all revolutionary efforts were stopped. Literature, philosophy and social concepts now evinced revanchist tendencies; for medicine this meant a general return to traditionalism and eclecticism. A look at the lecture lists of the universities shows that not only Brunonianism but the whole body of Romantic literature disappeared from the educational agenda.

But of course the ideas of this period were not lost. The generation of 1840 and after in its turn attacked the "intellectually barren time of medical eclecticism" and recalled the "revolutionary" ideas of "Romantic medicine" at the beginning of the century. For

[21] Tsouyopoulos, op. cit., note 3 above, pp. 173–6.

[22] Andreas Röschlaub, *Neues Magazin für die clinische Medizin,* Nuremberg, 1816.

[23] Georges Canguilhem, *On the normal and the pathological,* trans. Carolyn R. Fawcett, Studies in the History of Modern Science vol. 3, Dordrecht, Boston, and London, D. Reidel, 1978, pp. 24–7; see also Jean-François Braunstein, *Broussais et le matérialisme. Médecine et philosophie au XIXe siècle,* Paris, Meridiens Klincksieck, 1986; Nelly Tsouyopoulos, 'Die Erregungstheorie in Frankreich (Brownianismus auf den Kopf gestellt)', *Hist. Philos. Life Sci.,* 1989, **11:** 41–6; and Schwanitz, op. cit., note 13 above, pp. 102–3.

[24] Röschlaub, op. cit., note 22 above, pp. 153–90.

example, Wunderlich, a founder of thermometry in Germany and a protagonist of the new, so-called "physiological medicine" school in the 1840s, ascribed the genesis of this school to Brown and Röschlaub.[25]

In 1846, Bernard Hirschel, a German doctor and historian, published a study of Brunonianism.[26] He presented the subject very generally, and undertook the discussion of all aspects of the new doctrine. He judged the work of Brown and Röschlaub very favourably and also listed the relevant literature in a bibliography which remains the best compilation on this subject. The relative objectivity of this study also shows that, by then, John Brown was already considered a purely historical figure.

II

I shall try now to explain the phenomenon of Brown's reception in Germany and, to begin with, why the interest in him began at such a late date.

For the Germans, Brunonianism was not interesting as long as it was thought to be a mechanical theory similar to Haller's theory of irritability.[27] Brown's adages that "Life is a forced state" or "the tendency of animals' every moment is toward dissolution . . . they are kept from it by foreign powers",[28] were understood to suggest that organisms must be totally passive in the face of natural influences. Thus Brown's medical theory was categorized as one of the dogmatic theories, hostile to life and static at a time when German physiology had begun to embrace the ideas of evolution and progression in nature. Even Schelling at first rejected Brown's doctrines because, as he wrote, "Brown thinks of animal life as something totally passive, which is impossible".[29] Thus the general opinion was that Brown destroyed the independence and quality of life, introducing a barren principle according to which "life is always stimulated from outside", as the historian Eble summarized it.[30]

It was Röschlaub's interpretation which made Brown's principle acceptable. Röschlaub explained Brown's "excitability" as follows: organisms possess intrinsic activity, but this has no actual reality unless the organism is stimulated from the outside. Therefore individual organisms do not exist without stimulation; but as long as they are stimulated, they are able to develop more than a purely receptive reaction to stimuli.[31] Excitability is the basic capacity (or energy) inherent in, or given to, living matter. Life as such is only produced when outside influences act upon the excitability; but the response to the external stimulants is the combined product of both stimuli and excitability.[32]

[25] Owsei Temkin, 'Wunderlich, Schelling and the history of medicine', *Gesnerus*, 1966, **23**: 188–95.

[26] Bernard Hirschel, *Geschichte des Brownschen Systems und der Erregungstheorie*, Dresden and Leipzig, 1846.

[27] See Röschlaub's comments on the fifth chapter of the *Elementa* in op. cit., note 7 above, vol. 1, p. 49. See also Richard Toellner, 'Mechanismus-Vitalismus: ein Paradigmawechsel? Testfall Haller', in Alwin Diemer (editor), *Die Struktur wissenschaftlicher Revolutionen und die Geschichte der Wissenschaften*, Meisenheim am Glan, Hain, 1977; and Schwanitz, op. cit., note 13 above, pp. 65–6.

[28] *Elementa* I: lxxii; in Röschlaub, op. cit., note 7 above, vol. 1, p. 58.

[29] Schelling, op. cit., note 17 above, p. 506.

[30] Burkard Eble, *Die Geschichte der praktischen Arzneikunde. (Systeme, Epidemien, Heilmittel, Bäder) vom Jahre 1800–1825*, Vienna, 1840, p. 17.

[31] Röschlaub, op. cit., note 9 above, vol. 1, p. 244.

[32] Ibid., p. 238. See also Tsouyopoulos, op. cit., note 3 above, pp. 120–8; John Neubauer, 'Dr. John Brown (1735–88) and early German Romanticism', *J. Hist. Ideas*, 1967, **28**: 367–82; and Guenter B. Risse, 'The Brownian system of medicine: its theoretical and practical implications', *Clio Medica*, 1970, **5**: 45–51, p. 45.

Furthermore, Röschlaub differentiated Brown's excitability, saying that diseases were not brought about by a mere excess or lack of stimuli, but that these came about through a disproportion between the receptive and active constituents of excitability.[33] Schelling, accepting this interpretation of Röschlaub, changed his mind about Brown's doctrine. Brown, he wrote, "had elaborated the only true principles for the whole organic *Naturlehre* because he was the first to understand that life is neither absolutely passive nor absolutely active". And Schelling added: "Most partisans did not understand the scientific meaning of Brown's principles, . . . with one exception, Röschlaub, whose works everyone who has a sense for scientific medicine must study".[34]

Personal and psychological motives played an important role in the rapid reception of Brunonianism in Germany. Röschlaub's sudden fame, arising out of his advocacy of John Brown's doctrines, was certainly a great challenge to most physicians and intellectuals. Because Marcus was already one of the most renowned practitioners and director of the best hospital in Germany, his enthusiasm for Brown was very helpful, and, finally, Schelling's interest and co-operation made the movement attractive to circles outside medicine. Excitability theory thus became an essential part of German culture and therefore most people felt that they had to participate in the debates concerning it.[35] The translation of Brown's works into German helped to spread his ideas and contributed to his popularity.

A further question which I have to put now is: what were the German physicians seeking? What did they find, or think to find, in Brown's doctrines?

It is obvious from medical writings from around 1800 that medical professionals were not satisfied with the medical system in Germany and that they were trying to reform it.[36] Their main problem was the fact that they did not have a scientifically-based therapeutics. This problem was related to the physicians' economic and social status: doctors criticizing the medical system were mainly complaining about the low esteem in which their own profession was held. Even at the beginning of the nineteenth century, medical doctors in Germany were a minority among the healing practitioners. A doctor who did not succeed in finding employment with the state authorities could scarcely compete with such other healing professionals as surgeons, barbers, *Bademeister,* and quacks tolerated by the authorities.[37] Most people preferred the non-doctors, well established by tradition and, of course, much cheaper.

The doctors' main concern was to attain protection through the state. But the most thoughtful among them came to the conclusion that it would be difficult to demand protection against quackery from the authorities if regular medicine itself was not able to distinguish between genuine medical practice on the one hand and blind empiricism and quackery on the other. Röschlaub was convinced that Brown's ideas could give a

[33] Röschlaub, op. cit., note 9 above, vol. 1, pp. 237–47.

[34] Schelling, op. cit., note 18 above, p. 91. See also Tsouyopoulos, op. cit., note 18 above, pp. 107–17.

[35] See also Schwanitz, op. cit., note 13 above, pp. 92–3.

[36] Nelly Tsouyopoulos, 'Reformen am Bamberger Krankenhaus—Theorie und Praxis der Medizin um 1800', *Hist. Hospitalium,* 1976, **11**: 103–22. See also Urban Wiesing, *Umweltschutz und Medizinalreform in Deutschland am Anfang des 19. Jahrhunderts,* Cologne, Pahl-Rugenstein, 1987, pp. 53–68.

[37] Tsouyopoulos, op. cit., note 3 above, pp. 77–84.

scientific foundation to medicine, and thus help orthodox medicine to develop methods which could not be used by non-educated practitioners.[38]

Now why would John Brown's system, which was generally thought to be empirical, appear to the eyes of the Germans as a basis for scientific medicine? Central to any answer was Brown's idea that health and disease are identical.[39] This simple statement was important because it means that pathology, nosology, and clinical medicine could be linked to physiology, which was in turn considered to be a field to which the experimental methods of physics and chemistry were applicable. Scientific physiology was a part of medical education in Germany and every doctor knew about Haller's experiments concerning the life principles "irritability" and "sensibility"; but they could not see how they could use these basic sciences in the treatment of diseases.

Investigators had tried to establish a scientific pathology by linking it to physiology and deriving the pathogenesis of diseases from life principles. They had tried to prove that fever, inflammations, and tumours were due to qualitative or quantitative deviations from "normal" irritability and sensibility of the nerves and muscles. When they did not suceed, pathologists as well as clinicians began to doubt if the principles of physiology and the methods of mechanism and reductionism could help develop a scientific pathology.

And now excitability, according to John Brown, was a physiological principle which at the same time explained asthenia and sthenia as basic pathological states of the organism. It was a principle which seemed to solve the immediate problem; this aspect of Brunonianism, which impressed German intellectual physicians from the beginning,[40] was elucidated for the first time in this context in 1795, in Röschlaub's dissertation on fever. Röschlaub's thesis challenged the opinions of the established medical professionals, causing a controversy in the medical faculty.[41] Schelling, writing in the *Erster Entwurf* about the concept of the new scientific medicine, also primarily emphasized this aspect of the Brunonian principle.[42]

This reaction of German physicians to Brown's principle of excitability had already been prepared by the philosophy of Kant and Fichte. As I have already mentioned, the physicians' problems were not primarily philosophical. But as the establishment of scientific medicine became more difficult, they could not avoid the influence of philosophy. Kant's philosophy had remained authoritative for intellectual and social considerations in Germany; and physicians trying to attain a scientific status for medicine naturally took it as a starting point. In several papers Guenter Risse has shown which aspects of Kant's epistemology attracted physicians.[43] It is obvious that this ideal of how science should be was, in fact, a result of the critical philosophy of Kant.

[38] Röschlaub presented these ideas mainly in his book *Über Medizin ihr Verhältnis zur Chirurgie nebst Materialien zu einem Entwurfe der Polizei der Medizin*, Frankfurt, 1802.

[39] *Elementa*, II: ii; in Röschlaub, op. cit., note 7 above, vol. 2, pp. 140–1.

[40] Tsouyopoulos, op. cit., note 3 above, pp. 113–16.

[41] Andreas Röschlaub, *De febri fragmentum*, Bamberg, 1795. See also Tsouyopoulos, op. cit., note 3 above, p. 116.

[42] Schelling, op. cit., note 18 above, p. 230.

[43] 'Kant, Schelling and the early search for a philosophical "science" of medicine in Germany', *J. Hist. Med.*, 1972, **27**: 145–58; ' "Philosophical" medicine in nineteenth-century Germany: an episode in the relation between philosophy and medicine', *J. Med. & Philos.*, 1976, **1**: 72–91.

At the beginning of the 1790s the physicians' initial enthusiasm changed, however, to scepticism. They realized that medicine could not fulfill the conditions for Kantian science.[44] A "true" science, according to Kant, requires *a priori* principles from which empirical propositions are derived. Now Kant also made it clear which concepts could be used as *a priori* principles: namely, only those which have a mathematical structure. Such metaphysical concepts as "God" or "soul" lost their explanatory power. Also, of course, the famous life principle of the German tradition, the *Lebenskraft,* lost its rights as an *a priori* principle which could explain the phenomenon of life. And then Röschlaub suggested that John Brown's "excitability" concept could be used as an *a priori* principle to explain life and disease, without the epistemological difficulties to which other metaphysical concepts lead.[45]

Now what made Röschlaub and others believe this? Possibly it was the influence of Fichte's philosophy. I think that this sudden openness to the ideas of John Brown after 1795 is not entirely accidental. In 1794, Fichte's *Wissenschaftslehre* appeared, and in the following years the intellectual atmosphere was dominated by discussions about Fichte's work.[46] It was the poet Novalis who insisted that Brown's "excitability" was very similar to Fichte's *Wissenschaftslehre.*[47] Historians have found this comparison fatuous, but it was meaningful for people like Novalis, Röschlaub, and Schelling. Fichte's *Wissenschaftslehre* tried to establish a relationship between two heterogeneous beings (as subject and object), thereby avoiding the difficulties of both realism and idealism. This appeared similar to the problem German medicine had, in finding a relationship between organism (subject) and environment (object) which would avoid the difficulties of both mechanism and vitalism.

John Neubauer, commenting on Novalis's opinion on Fichte and Brown, added that both Fichte and the author of the *Elements of medicine* would certainly have protested against this analogy.[48] This may be true, but it is not important. Whether it was Brown's intention or not, through the influence of his ideas German medicine was able to formulate a "dialectical" relation between organism and environment, avoiding the difficulties of mechanism and vitalism; it was analogous to the relationship which Fichte elaborated between the "I" and "not I" at the level of consciousness.

Brown, like Fichte, saw the response of organisms to outside agents as a quantitative reaction which is equal to the stimuli. This response, which Brown called "excitement", is a life force separating the organic from the inorganic realm.[49] The essential point is that the excitement does not represent only the stimulation, but a combination of the

[44] See Erna Lesky, 'Cabanis und die Gewissheit der Heilkunst', *Gesnerus,* 1954, **11**: 152–82; and Tsouyopoulos, op. cit., note 3 above, pp. 180–4.

[45] Röschlaub, op. cit., note 9 above, vol. 1, pp. 103–207.

[46] Johann Gottlieb Fichte, *Über den Begriff der Wissenschaftslehre oder der sogenannten Philosophie als Einleitungsschrift zu seinen Vorlesungen über die Wissenschaft,* Weimar, 1794; *Grundlage der gesammten Wissenchaftslehre,* Weimar, 1794–5.

[47] 'Fichtes Wissenschaftslehre ist die Theorie der Erregung', in *Novalis' Schriften,* im Verein mit Richard Samuel hrsg. von Paul Kluckhohn, 4 vols., Leipzig, 1929, vol. 3, p. 383. See Neubauer, op. cit., note 32 above; and *idem,* 'Novalis und die Ursprünge der romantischen Bewegung in der Medizin', *Sudhoffs Archiv,* 1969, **53**: 160–70.

[48] *Idem,* op. cit., note 32 above, p. 376.

[49] *Elementa,* I: ii, iii; in Röschlaub, op. cit., note 7 above, vol. 1, pp. 5–7, 9–10. See also Risse, op. cit., note 32 above, p. 45.

stimulation and intrinsic excitability; thus, living matter has a basic capacity to perceive environmental impressions and to respond to them. In other words, the response of organisms to the environment is mediated by an intrinsic activity of the organism. At this point, according to the German interpretation, Brunonianism could be distinguished from all mechanical theories of life.[50]

Now what, in particular, distinguished Brunonianism from vitalistic theories? If excitability is a hypothetical capacity that cannot be directly experienced, then how is it different from such vital forces as *Lebenskraft* and *Bildungstrieb,* that were considered to be *causae occultae*?

Brown's excitability is not a *causa occulta* because it is no *causa* at all. The real cause of the visible excitement remains the outside stimulant. What Brown assumed was that a deficient stimulation, which is visible in a low degree of excitement, must leave great amounts of the intrinsic activity of the organism unused; on the other hand, excessive stimulation, reflected in a high degree of excitement, finally leads to a dangerous exhaustion of the amount of intrinsic activity (excitability). Both states indicate an imbalance in the organism that leads to disease.[51]

This formula, according to which excitability suffers opposite variations to the stimuli and the visible excitement, made Brown's principle verifiable, and as such applicable to practical medical diagnosis and therapy.[52] A practical consequence of this is, for example, the distinction between a direct asthenic state and the state that Brown called "indirect debility". In the latter, all vital expressions of the organism reflect over-abundance of excitement, produced by excessive external stimulation. Traditional medicine treated these cases mainly through blood-letting, trying to calm the high degree of excitement of the vital phenomena.[53] But according to Brunonianism, the physician must be aware of the fact that even if all vital phenomena reflect over-abundance of excitement, the organism can be extremely weak because its intrinsic capacity of reaction, its "resistance", is dangerously exhausted and therefore must be supported.[54]

Brown's "excitability" could thus be differentiated from other vitalistic theories. To German philosophers and physicians, "excitability" appeared to be a dialectic principle,[55] that could explain life and death, health and disease, and also the interaction between organisms and their environment.

The high expectations which the Germans invested in the excitability theory soon demanded a more precise explanation of its main principle. As we have seen, Röschlaub had already taken the first step in this direction. He considered excitability

---

[50] Röschlaub, op. cit., note 9 above, vol. 1, pp. 239–40; Schelling, op. cit., note 18 above, pp. 90–1.

[51] *Elementa,* II: iii; in Röschlaub, op. cit., note 7 above, vol. 1, pp. 9–36; see also Risse, op. cit., note 32 above, p. 46.

[52] Andreas Röschlaub, *Von dem Einflusse der Brown'schen Theorie in die praktische Heilkunde,* Würzburg, 1798; see also Tsouyopoulos, op. cit., note 3 above, pp. 108–16.

[53] Wiesing, op. cit., note 36 above, pp. 53–68.

[54] *Elementa* II: iii; in Röschlaub, op. cit., note 7 above, vol. 2, pp. 142–50; see also Risse, op. cit., note 32 above, p. 46.

[55] "Das dritte System setzt den Organismus als Subjekt und Objekt, Thätigkeit und Receptivität zugleich, und eben diese Wechselbestimmung der Receptivität und der Thätigkeit in Einen Begriff gefasst, ist nichts anderes als was Brown Erregbarkeit genannt hat". Schelling, op. cit., note 18 above, p. 90.

71

(*Erregbarkeit*) to be a synthetic concept consisting of two antithetical factors, receptivity and activity. Health and disease depend on the balance or imbalance of these two factors.[56]

But even Röschlaub's formulation did not satisfy Schelling, who put two further questions.[57] How can we explain the qualitative changes in an organism which also belong to the disease? and why does a certain degree of excitability mean health while a degree higher or lower mean disease? Sthenia and asthenia as states of disease made no sense, according to Schelling, unless what was meant by a "normal amount of excitability" was explained.[58] This could be done through the following hypothesis: every individual organism reproduces itself continuously. This process of self-reproduction is what we call life.[59] Every individual organism requires for its reproduction a special rhythm, and also needs for this purpose a certain degree of receptivity and an analogous degree of activity.[60] That is why every disproportion between the two factors of excitability means disease: because it disturbs the rhythm of self-reproduction and finally influences the reproduction process itself, thus causing not only quantitative but also qualitative changes in the organism. This was Schelling's major contribution to the medical theory of excitability. The explanation was adapted by Röschlaub and it soon became an essential part of medical theory in Germany.

Ordinary practitioners who were influenced by Brunonianism, or impressed by the success of Brunonian doctors, did not care so much about the new principles on which medical theory could be based. The only thing they understood was the fact that they had to change the treatment, and instead of calming the symptoms of high excitement by blood-letting and similar methods, they now recommended strengthening medication, and especially the administration of opium. It is understandable that abuse could not always be avoided; some practitioners used opium as a universal remedy and this fact became a major criticism against Brown and the whole movement.[61] Actually the abuse of new medical remedies was not much different from practices today; but at the beginning of the nineteenth century it was still possible to criticize such abuses successfully.

After a time, educated doctors in Germany became disappointed with Brunonianism, and even Röschlaub became sceptical. He did not reject Brown's medical theory, but he realized that the criteria for its application were not sufficient for the foundation of a scientific clinical medicine.[62] But even if Brunonianism did not give the German physicians what they expected for the reform of the medical system, the influence of Brown's ideas on German medical thought cannot be denied. Several characteristic and important new ideas of nineteenth-century medical thought cannot

[56] Röschlaub, op. cit., note 9 above, vol. 1, pp. 237–8.

[57] Schelling, op. cit., note 18 above, pp. 220–40 ('Theorie der Krankheit, abgeleitet aus der dynamischen Stufenfolge in der Natur').

[58] Ibid., p. 222.

[59] Ibid., p. 235.

[60] Ibid., p. 236.

[61] See Verena Jantz, 'Pharmacologia Browniana. Pharmakotherapeutische Praxis des Brownianismus aufgezeigt und interpretiert an den Modellen von A. F. Marcus in Bamberg und J. Frank in Wien', diss., Philipps-Universität Marburg, 1974; Hans-Uwe Lammel, 'Nosologische und therapeutische Konzeptionen in der romantischen Medizin', diss., Humboldt Universität, Berlin, 1986, pp. 142–4.

[62] *Neues Magazin,* op. cit., note 22 above, pp. 20–35.

be understood without the direct or indirect influence of John Brown's doctrines:[63] examples are the ideas that pathology cannot be considered identical to physiology unless one applies a quantitative concept of disease; and that quantitative concepts in medicine must express a proportional relationship (a synthesis of two factors). Related to this idea was a new concept of fever as a measurable, disproportionate organic reaction. Another Brunonian legacy was the idea that if nosology were used as a basis for diagnosis it must be dynamically conceived, namely as pathogenic and not as a static classificatory system.

But most influential of all was Brown's principle of excitability. After Brown and the Romantics, German medicine never returned to the pure mechanism of the eighteenth century. The idea of an active, self-reproducing and self-defending power mediating the organism's general reaction has, since then, never ceased to resonate in German medical thinking. This can be seen, for example, in Rudolf Virchow, especially when he was trying to formulate the general principles of cellular pathology.[64] He finally succeeded in establishing what Röschlaub had envisaged: a pathological method, the understanding and application of which distinguished doctors from other practitioners. Even today, medicine cannot avoid questions derived from the principle of excitability. Must physicians treat the reaction of the organism to external stimulation, or is it possible to support the self-repairing power of the organism? Can medicine support the self-regulating capacity of the organism as such?

The answer to these questions is as negative as it was in the nineteenth century. It is true that some concepts of Brunonianism and of the Romantics, like the psychosomatic concept of disease, or the dialectical interaction between organism and environment, are very attractive today, but the central idea of excitability cannot be more than an explanatory challenge. It remains one of the possibilities that scientific medicine, today totally based on reductionism, cannot accept. Thus the first goal of Brown and the Romantics does not coincide with the aims of the modern scientific community.

Positivistic historians of medicine found themselves in great difficulties trying to present the personalities of Brown, Röschlaub, and Schelling and to judge their role in the history of medicine. Aware of their great influence and of their ideas on the one hand, but also quite certain that they do not deserve a place among the heroes of scientific progress, historians judged them ingenious but mistaken, and concluded that they had hindered progress. Therefore they were given the honour of placement among the most prominent enemies of modern scientific medicine. In this respect positivistic historiography agrees with Goethe, who also bestowed on Schelling, Brown, and Röschlaub the honour of putting them in the pantheon of his enemies:[65]

---

[63] See also Schwanitz, op. cit., note 13 above, pp. 100–3.

[64] He wrote for example in his article 'Alter und neuer Vitalismus': "In der letzten Zeit hat man sich mehr an die functionelle Reizbarkeit (*irritabilitas*) gehalten . . .; ich habe daneben auch die nutritive und reproductive Reizbarkeit oder Erregbarkeit (*excitabilitas*) als eine mehr allgemein vitale Eigenschaft wieder zu begründen gesucht". *Arch. path. Anat. Physiol.* [Berlin], 1856, **9**: 3–55, p. 52.

Wenn ich nun im holden Haine
Unter meinen Freunden wandle,
Mögen's meine Feinde haben,
Die als Kegel ich behandle.

Kommt nur her, geliebte Freunde!
Lasst uns schleudern, lasst uns schieben;
Seht nur, es ist jedem Kegel
Auch sein Name angeschrieben.

Da den *Procerem* der Mitte
Tauft'ich mir zu Vater *Kanten*,
Hüben *Fichte*, drüben *Schelling*,
Als die nächsten Geistsverwandten.

Brown steht hinten in dem Grunde,
Röschlaub aber trutzt mir vorne,
Und besonders diesen letzten
Hab'ich immer auf dem Korne.

Dann die *Schlegels* und die *Tiecke*
Sollen durcheinander stürzen
Und durch ihre Purzelbäume
Mir die lange Zeit verkürzen.

---

[65] *Goethes Werke, herausgegeben im Auftrage der Grossherzogin Sophie von Sachsen,* vol. 5, pt. 1, Weimar, 1893, p. 167:

> When, surrounded by my friends,
> In goodly groves I sally,
> My enemies take on the guise
> Of skittles in an alley.
>
> Come here, dear friends, and let's begin
> The bowling and the throwing.
> Can't you see, on every pin,
> A name is clearly showing?
>
> "Father Kant" have I baptized
> The overtowering kingpin.
> Left is Fichte, Schelling's right,
> The closest of his mind's kin.
>
> Brown's behind, while at the front
> Röschlaub glowers impassive.
> Just the one at which to aim
> My retribution massive.
>
> Then the Schlegels and the Tiecks
> Shall knock down one another,
> And with their somersaultings end,
> This long and tiresome bother.
>
> *V.N.*

Medical History, Supplement No. 8, 1988, 75–88.

THE BRUNONIAN INFLUENCE ON THE MEDICAL THOUGHT AND PRACTICE OF JOSEPH FRANK

by

RAMUNAS KONDRATAS*

In Europe at the end of the eighteenth century and the beginning of the nineteenth a significant change was taking place in the perception, description, definition, and ordering of medical knowledge. Many physicians realized that medical knowledge could not be organized or ordered around a few basic principles or laws like mathematics or the physical sciences, nor could diseases be classified in the same manner as botanical or zoological species. Disease began to be perceived and described in terms of organic lesions rather than just symptoms. Pathological alterations of organs and tissues were studied by means of post-mortem examinations. New diagnostic techniques, such as auscultation and percussion, revealed structural changes in the body while the patient was still alive. Traditional observations gave way to clinical examination. The clinic and teaching hospital emerged as the important institutional settings for the study of diseases.

Much of the secondary literature on the history of clinical medicine at that time, such as the work of Ackerknecht and Foucault, has concentrated on the Paris school.[1] A comparative look at clinical medicine in different social and scientific contexts might lead to better generalizations about the nature of clinical medicine and its development.

Except for a very brief stay at the University of Göttingen, which was then under English rule, Johann Peter Frank (1745–1821) and his son Joseph Frank (1771–1842) spent all their lives working in absolutist states—the Holy Roman and Russian Empires.[2] Together they taught at the universities of Pavia, Vienna, and Vilnius. In

* Dr Ramunas Kondratas, Curator, Medical Sciences Division, National Museum of American History, Smithsonian Institution, Washington DC 20560, USA.

[1] E. H. Ackerknecht, *Medicine at the Paris Hospital 1794–1848*, Baltimore, Johns Hopkins University Press, 1967; M. Foucault, *The Birth of the clinic*, trans. A. M. Sheridan Smith, New York, Pantheon Books, 1973. In recent years there have been more attempts at comparative analyses of the development of clinical medicine, such as O. Keel, 'The politics of health and the institutionalization of clinical practices in Europe in the second half of the eighteenth century', in W. F. Bynum and R. Porter (editors), *William Hunter and the eighteenth-century medical world*, Cambridge University Press, 1985, pp. 207–56.

[2] The most complete and accurate biographical information about the Franks is contained in their unpublished memoirs, 'Mémoires biographiques de Jean Pierre Frank, et de Joseph Frank, son fils, rédigés par ce dernier', MS, University of Vilnius Library, Lithuanian SSR, 5 vols., (Leipzig, 1848). Unless noted otherwise, all of my biographical data will be taken from this source and cited as *Mémoires biographiques*. The Roman numeral denotes the volume number, followed by the chapter number and the page(s). The manuscript pages have been numbered twice and I will give both page citations. An abridged Polish translation of the memoirs was published by W. Zahorski, *Pamiętniki*, 3 vols., Vilnius, Księgarnia Stowarz. naucz. polskiego, 1921. A few excerpts from the memoirs were published, in the original French, in several journals by S. Trzebiński during the 1920s. Some biographical materials relating to Johann Peter Frank have been translated and published by George Rosen, 'Biography of Dr. Johann Peter Frank . . . written by

addition, Johann Peter Frank was the director of the Medical-Surgical Academy in St Petersburg. As medical thinkers and writers; as medical organizers and reformers; as personal physicians and councillors of state to princes, emperors, and tsars; and as directors of major hospitals and founders of several clinics, medical societies, and institutes in both Western and Eastern Europe, they played an important role in the development of clinical medicine. They travelled extensively and were personally acquainted with many of the major physicians and scientists in Western and Eastern Europe as well as with the work of the leading medical and scientific institutions in those countries. The evolution of their medical ideas and the thrust of their medical reforms closely reflected many of the transformations occurring in medicine at the end of the eighteenth century and the beginning of the nineteenth.

The medical ideas of John Brown played an important role in shaping the thought and practice of Joseph Frank, and it is this encounter that I shall describe in this paper.[3] Frank's experience with the Brunonian doctrine went full circle: from initial adherence and adulation to moderate skepticism and then, finally, to rejection, not only of Brunonianism but of medical systems in general.

The intellectual milieu in which the medical thought of Joseph Frank developed, and which predisposed him to the ideas of Brown, consisted of many intertwined themes. Most of them, when teased out, reveal an ancient ancestry and a preoccupation with the definition of medicine in relation to other intellectual endeavours and practices, especially the natural sciences. There were such recurrent themes as the search for order and certainty, mechanism vs. vitalism, empiricism vs. rationalism, general disease states vs. specific diseases, and science vs. art. At the end of the eighteenth century, these themes were interpreted within the conceptual framework of the French philosophy of Ideology, German *Naturphilosophie*, and British empiricism. In the course of his intellectual development, Joseph Frank was subjected to all of these influences.

The intimate relationship between medicine and the natural sciences is especially important for understanding medical thought because the natural sciences provided the leading paradigms and principles for the numerous medical systems of the eighteenth century.[4] Medical systems were formed around a small number of fundamental principles, at first drawn chiefly from mechanics but later also from chemistry, from which, by deductive reasoning, all clinical and therapeutic phenomena supposedly could be explained. Mechanistic philosophy, at the beginning of the century, as well as the discovery of new gases, electricity, and galvanism toward its

---

himself', *J. Hist. Med.,* 1948, **3**: 11–46, 279–314. The standard nineteenth-century biographical dictionaries also have entries on the Franks.

[3] Much of the material for this paper has been taken from chapters 4–6 of my 'Joseph Frank (1771–1842) and the development of clinical medicine: a study of the transformation of medical thought and practice at the end of the 18th and the beginning of the 19th centuries', Ph.D. diss., Harvard University, 1977. Brunonianism was the focus of my senior honours thesis, 'The Brunonian doctrine and Joseph Frank', Harvard University, 1970. Others who have analysed the influence of the Brunonian doctrine on Joseph Frank have been R. Müller, *Joseph Frank (1771–1842) und die Brownsche Lehre,* Zurich, Juris, 1970; and S. Trzebiński, 'Brownizm w świetle pamiętników Franka', [Brunonianism in the light of the Frank memoirs], *Archwm Hist. Filoz. Med.,* 1924, **1**: 113–26.

[4] There are many secondary sources concerning the medical systems of the eighteenth century, e.g., Lester King, *The medical world of the eighteenth century,* University of Chicago Press, 1958.

latter half exerted strong influences on medicine and inspired new medical systems.

Newtonian and Cartesian physics reinforced the notion of mathematical (geometric) reasoning and mechanism in medicine (the hydraulic model of physiological function), thereby giving further impetus to iatrophysics. Mechanical forces and dynamic principles formed the core of Friedrich Hoffmann's (1660–1742) medical system, which greatly influenced the work of such later systematists as Hieronymus Gaub (1705–90), William Cullen (1710–90), and John Brown. Their iatromechanical hypotheses tended to focus the attention of physicians on the solid parts of the body, the muscles and nerves. Health was defined in terms of a proper muscle-nerve tone. Changes in this tone—either spasms or atony—resulted in disease.

The experimental work of Albrecht von Haller (1708–77) on tissue irritability and sensibility further accelerated the shift away from the predominant doctrine of humours to solidist pathology. It also illustrated to many of his contemporaries that scientific methodology could be successfully applied to medicine, that properties of living matter analogous to those of inert matter could be discovered and described. The mechanistic interpretation of vital functions, the neural concept of disease, and the belief in vital forces analogous to physical forces were all notions that played an important role in forming Joseph Frank's early medical thought.

The medical system of Brown has been well described already. It addressed many of the major concerns of medicine in its day—the need for certainty, the need to relate medical theory and practice, the need to find a vital force or principle responsible for the organization of organic matter, and the need for medical reforms. The fact that it addressed these needs (rightly or wrongly) as well as its supposed novelty and simplicity largely explain its great appeal. Rudolf Virchow compared the stir caused by the publication of Brown's *Elements of medicine* in Edinburgh in 1780 to the effect of an earthquake which shook the whole European continent and even the physicians of the New World.[5]

From the medical point of view, the Brunonian doctrine did not contain much that was new; and its scientific value cannot compare with that of the work of Haller, Morgagni, or Bichat. Brunonian therapeutics were meant to be clear, simple, and mathematically precise. But medical practice could not be reduced to such mathematical simplicity or exact conditions, especially given the state of clinical and pharmacological knowledge at that time. Moreover, Brown's over-simplified system did not demand much knowledge of anatomy and did away with any qualitative considerations regarding body fibres and fluids. It ignored the symptoms, physical signs, and structural changes associated with disease, and rejected the correlation of bedside data (as well as anatomical lesions) with autopsy findings: "never expect to discover the cause of disease in dead bodies", wrote Brown.[6] In fact, the Brunonian doctrine opposed many of the major tenets of clinical medicine and pathological anatomy. Nevertheless, as the example of the Franks will show, it did attract the attention of clinicians and there were serious attempts to apply it in the clinic.

[5] G. Rath, 'Alexander von Humboldt and Brunonianism', *J. Hist. Med.*, 1960, **15**: 75–7, p. 75.

[6] *The works of Dr John Brown M.D. To which is prefixed a biographical account of the author, by W. C. Brown*, 3 vols., London, J. Johnson, 1804, vol. 2, para. 84, pp. 199–200.

Joseph Frank heard about John Brown during a journey to Switzerland in the summer of 1791.[7] In June of that year, at the age of 20, Joseph had received his medical degree from the University of Pavia, where his teachers had been Spallanzani, Volta, and Scarpa, and a month later he and his father departed for Switzerland.

Upon his return to Pavia, a close friend and colleague, Vincent Solenghi, asked him about the new things that he had learned about medicine on his journey. Among others, Joseph mentioned that he had heard about a physician Brown, who thought that he could cure all diseases with alcohol and opium. Solenghi replied that he was misinformed, that Brown was really a "great genius" who had tried to apply to medicine the philosophy of Bacon and Newton.[8] Since Solenghi at that time did not possess a copy of Brown's *Elements of medicine*, he recommended that Joseph read a book by Robert Jones, a pupil and follower of Brown, which described the philosophical basis of Brown's system. It was entitled *An inquiry into the state of medicine, on the principles of inductive philosophy* (London, 1781). Joseph and Solenghi spent the rest of the summer reading and discussing Jones's book, which touched on many of the important issues facing physicians then, particularly the questions concerning the certainty or scientificity of their craft.[9]

A strong impulse to improve medical practice motivated Joseph Frank, and other young physicians trained in different medical traditions, to examine seriously the tenets of the Brunonian doctrine. They were seeking a scientific base for medicine, a medical theory to guide clinical practice. The anti-humoral, solidist, and physiological medical system of Brown was new, simple, and short in every proposition. It avoided philosophizing about the cause of life and confined itself to explaining the phenomena that life produced. It was opposed to the prevailing doctrine of antiphlogistic or debilitating treatment of diseases—blood-letting and purgatives—and above all, according to its followers, it conferred upon medicine the character of a science by applying to medicine the philosophical principles of Bacon and Newton.

Although reading Jones's work and then that of Brown greatly inspired Joseph, he did not agree with all the comparisons that Jones made between Bacon and Brown. Some of Bacon's axioms, he found, were favourable to Brown's doctrine but many

[7] It is unclear when Joseph first heard about Brown's medical doctrine. A. Adomowicz (1802–81), an assistant to Joseph at the University of Vilnius, claimed that Joseph had heard about Brown "from the mouth of his father" and had "become so inspired that he wrote a little work in Italian in 1786 about the subject." See his 'Prof. Józef Frank i jego teorya lekarska', *Gazeta lekarska* [Warsaw], 1868, **5**: 72. In the *Gesundheitstaschenbuch für das Jahr 1801*, Vienna, 1801, it is mentioned that the Franks made a brief visit or stopover in Edinburgh in 1786 and a longer visit there from September 1789 to May 1790. On both occasions they would undoubtedly have heard about Brown. It is odd that neither trip was mentioned in either of the Franks' memoirs; both usually described their journeys in detail. Joseph briefly stated, in a published letter to Brugnatelli, that there were whispers in Pavia about Brown in 1790: *Über die Lehre von Brown an Herrn Brugnatelli*, trans. from the Italian by A. M. Weikard, Frankfurt, 1796, p. 26. So the chances are very good that Joseph had already heard something about Brown before going to Switzerland in 1791, even though the first mention of Brown in his memoirs is in connection with that trip (*Mémoires biographiques*, I. 23. 413/389).

[8] J. Frank, *Mémoires biographiques*, I. 23. 430/406. Also see J. Frank, 'Biographie du docteur John Brown', in *Médecine portative, ou guide de santé*, Paris, Pironnet, 1803, pp. 16–42. Here Frank described his early reading of, and experiences with, the Brunonian doctrine at Pavia.

[9] G. Risse has elaborated on this theme in 'The quest for certainty in medicine: John Brown's system of medicine in France', *Bull. Hist. Med.*, 1971, **45**: 1–12 and 'The Brownian system of medicine: its theoretical and practical implications', *Clio Medica*, 1970, **5**: 45–51.

others were contrary to it, as well as to all medical systems.[10] At this time he was more concerned with those axioms that were favourable. Yet he never lost sight of those that were objectionable. Eventually they would come to the forefront as he tried to apply the Brunonian doctrine in practice, and to reconcile it with new findings in the natural sciences.

Johann Peter was content to see Joseph so eagerly pursuing his studies and clinical practice. Thinking that his great enthusiasm for Brown would soon fade, he did not hinder him in any way. He noted that his students' preoccupation with the Brunonian theory increased both their enthusiasm and the accuracy of their clinical observations.[11] They began to pay more attention to the cause of disease, and to the effects of such external agents as food, drink, air, and drugs on the body. Brown was read "night and day". Some admired his doctrine for its novelty, while others were unable to accept it because they felt it led to great errors in treatment. Many debates ensued.

The fact that Johann Peter did not sharply attack the Brunonian doctrine and even defended Joseph's sympathy to it, explains in part the good reception that Brown's ideas received in Italy. Nevertheless, Johann Peter cautioned his students against blindly accepting the doctrine of Brown. He felt that he did not understand well all of Brown's ideas and thus did not want either to defend him, or accuse him of some grievous error. But he did disagree with him in many respects and clearly articulated his points of disagreement. He also tried to show that many of the ideas that Brown claimed to be new, and his own, were really taken from others. In presenting his opinions and criticism, both to his students and in the press, Johann Peter tried to avoid bitter sectarian debates which would only leave bad feelings on both sides. This attitude, combined with the eclectic nature of his teaching, produced an atmosphere conducive to a critical examination of the Brunonian doctrine.

Joseph's earliest publications, panegyric in tone, were explanations of and commentaries on the works of Brown and his followers. His first publication, an Italian-language tract on the Brunonian system (1794), described Jones's work and commented on a number of other books written in Britain and Italy concerning the Brunonian doctrine. He ended by saying:

> I hope that this work will be received by the followers of Brown as a sign of my eagerness to fulfill their wishes and I am not concerned about their enemies among whom are many of my admired teachers.[12]

The following year he translated Jones's *Inquiry* into Italian, and appended his own notes concerning some of his earliest *practical* experiences with the Brunonian doctrine.[13] According to William Cullen Brown, the son of John Brown, Joseph was

---

[10] J. Frank, *Mémoires biographiqes,* I. 24. 434/410.

[11] Johann Peter described the reaction of his students to Brown and his own views on the Brunonian doctrine in his introduction to Joseph's *Heilart in der klinischen Lehranstalt zu Pavia,* trans. F. Schaeffer, Vienna, Camesina, 1797, pp. 19–29.

[12] Joseph Frank, *Über die Lehre,* op. cit., note 7 above, p. 70.

[13] J. Frank, *Ricerche sullo stato della medicina secondo i principi della filosofia indutiva,* 2 vols., Pavia, 1795.

"the most assiduous and successful in promoting the new principles of medicine".[14] But slowly, as Joseph's clinical experience increased, his views began to moderate. The clinics at Pavia and Vienna became his testing grounds.

When Joseph began his work at Pavia in 1792, he felt that he was very successful in applying Brown's principles at the bedside. The only exception was the case of a young girl suffering from typhus who was given 20 drops of laudanum, three times a day, fell into a deep coma and died. Nevertheless his apparent overall success encouraged other young physicians to ask Joseph for private lessons in the "new doctrine". Soon a small circle of approximately thirty persons was formed and began meeting regularly to discuss Brown's medical doctrine. Joseph agreed to meet with them, but on the condition that his father be kept ignorant of these meetings.

In order to avoid conflicts with the faculty, Joseph often had to mask his Brunonian views with what he called "ancient nomenclature". After he wrote the apologetic tract in Italian mentioned above, in 1794, his father angrily warned him that by publicly coming out in favour of Brown's system he would close off his own entry into the university and the hospital. The warning was very sound. Even though the university and the hospital were not completely closed to him (largely due to the reputation of his father), his Brunonianism did hinder his early career. As a medical assistant at the Pavia clinic and a repetitor of special therapy, he had to moderate or disguise his true beliefs while pursuing his academic duties. Two years later (1796), when he joined his father in Vienna, he was not allowed to teach at the university because of his Brunonian views and so had to give private lessons instead.[15]

When Johann Peter left for Vienna in 1795, Joseph took over the Pavia clinic and his father's course on special therapy. He kept his father informed about his work in the clinic and took every opportunity to bring up Brown's doctrine. An extract from one letter in particular reveals his strong feelings. In that letter he stated that the anatomist Antonio Scarpa at Pavia was inclined toward the Brunonian doctrine and that in time Johann Peter would also embrace it. He then mentioned several ways in which the views of Brown and his father were compatible. Joseph suggested that his father follow the example of the Irish chemist Richard Kirwan (1733–1812), who abandoned an early belief in phlogiston in order to embrace "the system of Lavoisier".[16]

In his clinical reports from Pavia, Joseph classified most of the diseases that he observed as asthenic, that is, due to lack of excitement.[17] The influence of Brown, who thought that most diseases were asthenic, is quite apparent. One of the difficulties in applying the Brunonian therapy in the clinic was that it denied any specific action of

---

[14] W.C. Brown, op. cit., note 6 above, vol. 1, p. 163.

[15] In Vienna, Joseph worked as a hospital physician at the Allgemeine Krankenhaus and helped to organize a Society of Physicians, which was very pro-Brunonian. For a brief description of Brunonianism in Vienna see E. Lesky, *The Vienna Medical School of the 19th century*, trans. L. Williams and T. S. Levij, Baltimore, Johns Hopkins University Press, 1976, pp. 8–12.

[16] J. Frank, *Mémoires biographiques*, I. 27. 505/461. For more information on Kirwan's transformation see Aaron J. Ihde, *The development of modern chemistry*, New York, Harper and Row, 1964, p. 81.

[17] Joseph published a collection of observations at the Pavia clinic entitled *Ratio instituti clinici Ticinensis a mense Januario usque ad finem Junii 1795*, with a preface by J. P. Frank, Vienna, Camesina, 1797, which was translated into German by F. Schaeffer that same year: see note 11, above.

drugs. Diseases were the result of certain imbalances in the stimuli causing a change in the general state of the body. Since Brown believed that most diseases were asthenic and thus in need of stimulating treatment, general weakness or debility was the predominant state of the diseased body. At Pavia, Joseph often used opium, Peruvian bark, camphor, alcohol, musk, and other stimulating drugs although to a much more moderate extent than did most Brunonians. His experiences in the clinic, especially the death of the young girl from typhus, showed him the negative consequences of the improper and immoderate use of those drugs.

But Joseph did not confine himself to the use of stimulating remedies. He attempted to cure oedema with digitalis; mental disorders with belladonna; and pneumonia, whooping cough, and asthma with seneca roots, ipecac, and tartar emetic. He couched the actions of the drugs within a Brunonian explanatory scheme by stating that these diseases were due to a general weakness of the body and that the drugs acted on this weakness by raising the excitement.[18] For example, oedema was explained as a general weakness of the body (asthenia), especially of those organs responsible for the separation of water. Digitalis excited the body in general and thus acted as a diuretic. Even though Joseph at this time still denied the specific actions of drugs, the fact that he used a large variety of drugs in his treatment already distinguished him from most other Brunonians.

Joseph modified (in many instances just moderated) the Brunonian doctrine in several different ways. Clinical experience had shown him that such infectious diseases as typhus, smallpox, measles, and scarlet fever followed a characteristic and unchanging course despite the administration of stimulants. The use of stimulating drugs in such cases could cause more harm than good.

The truth of this observation was really brought home to him by the tragic death in 1796 of his younger brother Francis from the petechial typhus he contracted while practising in the Vienna clinic. Francis, who had also been an ardent supporter of Brown, had received his medical degree from Pavia. Later he went to Vienna together with Johann Peter and worked as one of his assistants in the Allgemeine Krankenhaus, the General Hospital. Joseph described his death as "one of the most terrible catastrophes of my life".[19] A few days after treating a case of petechial typhus, Francis began feeling very ill. He started taking Dover's powder, which contained ipecac and made him sweat, but to no avail. When he felt himself grow weaker, he began drinking Malaga wine and taking quinine (Peruvian bark). This resulted in a strong diarrhoea, which he treated with opium. Diarrhoea gave way to other nervous symptoms for which he took musk, camphor, blisters, and hot baths, but all in vain. The public, and even some physicians, attributed his death to the Brunonian method.[20] Regardless of the different speculations concerning causes of Francis's death, the fact remains that it had a very sobering effect upon Joseph's Brunonianism.

[18] The therapy employed by Joseph in the Pavia clinic has been analysed in greater detail by F. Aicher, 'Der Einfluss der Brownschen Lehre auf die Therapie. Untersucht an den von Frank im Krankenhaus zu Pavia behandelten Krankheiten', diss., University of Munich, 1933.

[19] J. Frank, *Mémoires biographiques*, I. 28. 545/495.

[20] Ibid., I. 28. 546/496–547/497. This was not the first or only death of a young physician at the General Hospital from what had been called "nosocomial typhus". In fact, several later observers remarked about the poor sanitary conditions and uncleanliness at the General Hospital. See Coste, 'Hôpital', *Dictionaire*

Shortly after Francis's death, Napoleon's army entered Pavia and the university was closed. Joseph had left just before its arrival to join his father in Vienna. There he continued to play an active role in propagating the Brunonian doctrine by organizing a group of young medical men into a private medical society similar to the one in Pavia. In his hospital and clinical practice he was particularly preoccupied with the treatment of febrile diseases, especially typhus. No doubt the death of Francis and others had focused his attention on this disease. In his writings, he began to re-analyse the principles of Brown's doctrine in the light of his clinical experience. He wanted to correct those principles that he could, reject those that were false, and, most importantly, pick out the most doubtful ones and make them the objects of further study.

In contrast with Brown, whose position was ambiguous, Joseph considered excitability to be a property of matter, which manifested itself in different ways depending on the material composition of the organs. Thus excitability could become irritability in the muscle, and sensibility in the nerve. Since excitability was identified with matter and could be expressed differentially in the body fabric, the structural organization of the different organs was important. Because organs differed in their function and organization, drugs would affect each of them differently. Diseases with such different characteristics could not all arise from one cause, namely asthenia or weakness.[21]

This was a major departure from Brown, who denied that there could be any kind of *qualitative* changes associated with excitability. Differences in the way stimuli affected excitability were purely *quantitative* and thus subject to mathematical analysis. Joseph ignored Brown's exact mathematical calculations of excitability and called the degree chart "nonsense". For him, the important criterion in choosing drugs was the diseased organ or organ system.

We thus see Joseph slowly starting to take the steps which would soon disengage him from the monistic concept that all diseases could be viewed as the result of variations in a single property or force, such as excitability. Even though he still closely linked vitality (or life) with a single force or property, the stress that he placed on the importance of organization would eventually lead him closer to the idea that vitality might be associated with that organization, that by means of organization the living being could be distinguished from the non-living. This became a major theme or metaphor of biochemical thought in the late eighteenth and early nineteenth centuries as described by Figlio, Jacob, and others.[22] The general orientation of

---

des sciences médicales, eds. F. P. Chaumeton and F. V. Mérat de Vaumartoise, Paris, Panckoucke, vol. 21, 1818, pp. 466–544, and 'Some account of the General Hospital and Medical School at Vienna', *Edinb. Med. Surg. J.,* 1806, **2:** 491–6. Johann Peter himself warned the competent authorities that so many foreign physicians and surgeons were attending the clinical lectures that "all relation vanished between the space available in the clinic and the number of students". Rosen, op. cit., note 2 above, p. 305.

[21] A chart comparing the views of Brown and Frank on excitability can be found in the article 'Auch eine Geschichte des Brownschen Systems', *Journal der Erfindungen, Theorien und Widersprüche in der Natur und Arzneiwissenschaft* [Gotha], 1796, **19:** 29–30.

[22] K. Figlio, 'The metaphor of organization: an historiographical perspective on the bio-medical sciences of the early nineteenth century,' *Hist. Sci.,* 1976, **14:** 17–53; F. Jacob, *The logic of life,* New York, Pantheon Books, 1973, pp. 74–129.

Joseph's work was clearly to the interior of the body, to its fabric or structure—a very important and necessary precondition for shifting or redirecting his attention to pathological anatomy. This shift was greatly accelerated by his journey, or "scientific voyage" as he called it, to Paris and London in 1802, where his faith in the Brunonian system, and systems in general, was totally shattered.

The new scientific ethos and ideas, especially the emphasis on rational empiricism, in France after the Revolution of 1789 and Great Britain during the Industrial Revolution played an important catalytic role in transforming his medical beliefs. Joseph was particularly influenced by the anti-Brunonian attitude of most of the leading physicians that he met. The advocates of Brunonianism, on the other hand, made a poor impression on him. Most of these he met in Germany on his way to Paris. Such pillars of German Brunonianism as Andreas Röschlaub, Adalbert Marcus, and Melchior Weikard, with whom he had eagerly collaborated in popularizing Brown's ideas, left a very bad impression. He used such terms as "scatter-brained", "conceited", "hypochondriac", and "misanthrope" to describe them.[23]

In Paris, where he met many dignitaries and important political figures including Napoleon I, Joseph spent most of his time visiting medical, scientific, and philanthropic institutions as well as discoursing with leading physicians and scientists.[24] The following list should serve to illustrate the breadth of his acquaintance with the eminent men of French science: Fourcroy, Monge, Berthollet, Chaptal, Laplace, Lacépède, Vauquelin, Guyton de Morveau, Portal, Lalande, Hallé, Pinel, Esquirol, Alibert, Richerand, Larrey, Desgenettes, and Corvisart.[25] These men were at the forefront, shaping the newly emergent French science and medicine: a science which placed particular emphasis on technology and the applied sciences, and a medicine of empirical observations. The sentiment against dogmatism, theorizing, and systematization was very strong.[26]

The French clinicians were particularly skeptical towards general theories and systems in medicine. They strongly attacked Joseph's Brunonianism. The ageing physician and surgeon Antoine Portal (1742–1832) said that he had read many of Joseph's works and that they filled him with both pleasure and pain:

> Pleasure because they showed proof that his talents would qualify him one day to take the place of his illustrious father; pain because he saw him bogged down in a system which, like the French constitution, was beautiful on paper but did not mean anything in practice.[27]

---

[23] J. Frank, *Mémoires biographiques,* II. 36. 181/195. Their work has been analysed in great detail by G. Risse, 'The history of John Brown's medical system in Germany during the years 1790–1806', PhD. diss., University of Chicago, 1971.

[24] For a description of the institutions that he visited see his *Reise nach Paris, London, und einem grossen Theile des übrigen Englands und Schottlands,* 2 vols., Vienna, 1804–5.

[25] Extracts from the memoirs describing Joseph's journey to Paris entitled 'Le séjour à Paris du Dr. Frank (1803)', have been published in *Bull. Soc. fr. d'Hist. Méd.,* 1924, **18**: 107–24.

[26] This sentiment was summarized nicely by A. F. Fourcroy, a leading spokesman of French science, who said that it was necessary to abandon systems and return to observation as a guide in the study of diseases. Antoine François de Fourcroy, (editor), *La médecine éclairée par les sciences physiques,* [etc.], Paris, Buisson, vol. 1, 1791, p. 142.

[27] 'Le séjour', op. cit., note 25 above, p. 112.

Hallé, Pinel, and Corvisart also criticized Joseph's Brunonian views; Corvisart in particular took great pleasure in "tormenting" him about Brown's system. The students at the Paris medical school were attracted to him because they had never seen a Brunonian and viewed him as a "curiosity". On leaving for London Joseph remarked that his "republican spirit" was entirely extinguished and that his Brunonianism was beginning "to totter".[28]

In Great Britain, the Industrial Revolution had a marked effect on British science. Scientific societies were formed in the new industrial towns. Philanthropic institutions were founded to take care of the sick, the poor, and the homeless. New clinics, hospitals, and vaccination institutes were built. In all the towns that Joseph visited, he first made the acquaintance of the leading physicians, then he went on a tour of the hospitals, clinics, philanthropic and scientific institutions, scientific societies, and prisons.[29] He was interested in seeing how various diseases were treated, how the medical and scientific institutions were organized and administered, and in hearing the ideas and opinions of his contemporaries on various medical subjects.

In Edinburgh he learned that Brown's doctrines had dazzled many students there, who had made use of them in writing their inaugural dissertations, but that all the professors were opposed to them. From Brown's son, William Cullen Brown, he learned about the circumstances surrounding the split between Cullen and Brown, and the numerous hardships and intrigues that Brown endured while in London. He saw the house in which Cullen had lived, and procured a consultation written in his hand. Cullen's memory as a practitioner, Joseph said, was greatly revered by the public of Edinburgh, but his theories had already been forgotten.[30] The new scientific ethos emerging in Great Britain was not conducive to the development of any general system of medicine, be it that of Cullen or Brown. Hypotheses and theories were to be based on experiment and observation. No one system could explain all the varied physiological and pathological phenomena. Thus the emphasis must be on treating individual diseases.

After leaving Bath, where he had visited Drs Falconer, Parry, and Haygarth, he proclaimed, "They have completed detaching me from the system of Brown."[31] And later, reflecting on his journey, he added, "I feel that I have been transformed into another man."[32] The "other man" of whom Joseph wrote was the one critical of systems and broad generalizations, the one who relied on correct diagnosis and treatment of each disease according to its particular requirements.

When Joseph returned to Vienna in December 1803, he had a series of conversations with his father which vividly revealed the transformation that had taken place in his thinking. Johann Peter had already surmised from Joseph's letters that his enthusiasm

---

[28] Ibid., p. 124.

[29] All of these institutions are described in his *Reise*. Extracts from his memoirs describing the many noted people that he met on this trip were published in the original French by S. Trzebiński in *Pamiętnik Wileńskiego Towarzystwa Lekarskiego*, 1929, **5**: z. 2, pp. 94–102, 200–7, 345–9 and 347–80.

[30] Ibid., pp. 203–4.

[31] Ibid., p. 206.

[32] Ibid., p. 207.

for Brown had waned, but did not know that he had completely renounced the Brunonian system. When Joseph finally made his declaration, Johann Peter was greatly distressed. He said,

> Why go from one extreme to the other? Modify as much as you like the principles which you defended with such ardour and success, but do not renounce them. One cannot teach the practice of medicine without arranging the facts related to that science in a certain order and then linking them together, that's what constitutes a system. That of Brown is defective, as I always told you, but the other systems are equally so. You have suffered so much for your Brunonianism, and now that one could call your victorious, you want to reverse your fortunes?

And Joseph answered,

> My dear father, I would very willingly follow your advice if I weren't convinced that it is precisely in the fundamental principles that the system of Brown is defective. I believe that they are incompatible with the practice of medicine based on experience. And why shouldn't I be able to arrange the result of this practice in some kind of order without subordinating it to a system? If I victoriously defended a cause as bad as Brunonianism, what success awaits me in defending rational empiricism, to which all physicians return sooner or later and which has been extolled by Hippocrates, Sydenham, Baglivi, and others?[33]

It was much easier, he said, to renounce the system of Brown, than to practise medicine at the bedside of the sick with it as a guide.

Joseph stayed in Vienna only eight months after his journey to Paris and London and then, together with his father, mostly for political reasons, left for the University of Vilnius in Lithuania, which was then a part of the Russian Empire. There Joseph worked for nearly 20 years and put into practice his "new" medical beliefs.

The first annual report of the Vilnius clinic, published in 1803, marked Joseph's formal break with the Brunonian system.[34] When discussing his earlier support of Brown he emphasized that he never completely agreed with all of Brown's ideas and that, on the contrary, he had brought to light and analysed several mistakes or false hypotheses made by Brown. He admitted that his biggest mistake was in thinking that all of medicine could be explained within the context of one system, and that he was ashamed of the "fetters" with which the love of this system had bound him. Observation and reason were now to be the base of his medical practice. Experience of the greatest physicians, observation of what kinds of treatment were most useful, and consideration of the climate and time of year were the medical principles according to which he was going to structure his practice. Thus, in his first clinical report from Vilnius, he described the medical topography of the Vilnius area and the diseases prevalent there during 1805–6. In his lectures on pathology and special therapeutics he used his father's textbook (*De curandis hominum morbis epitome*) and that of G. Borsieri (*The institutions of the practice of medicine*). He began making plans to write

---

[33] Ibid., pp. 378–9 (with corrections from the original manuscript of the memoirs).

[34] J. Frank, *Acta instituti clinici caesareae universitatis Vilnensis,* 3 vols., Leipzig, 1808–12. Volumes one and two were translated into German by J. Meyer as *Annalen des klinischen Instituts an der Kaiserlichen Universitaet zu Wilna,* Berlin, 1810, especially pp. 1–29. I disagree with the recent article by Bozena Plonka-Syroka, which argues that Joseph's break with Brunonianism occurred in 1822: 'Józef Frank i Jędrzej Śniadecki wobec doktryny Johna Browna', *Archwm Hist. Filoz. Med.,* 1986, **49**: 359–74.

his own medical textbook. The treatise that he envisioned certainly reflected the transformation that he had undergone:

> . . . I particularly have in mind a work confined to facts, with the exclusion of all hypotheses, unless they are mentioned in an historical account, or to show the errors to which the mania of wanting to explain everything can lead.[35]

Shortly before the first clinical report from Vilnius appeared in print, Joseph received a letter from Corvisart (dated 30 December 1807) with the following comment on Joseph's break with the Brunonian doctrine:

> I confess, from the bottom of my heart, that I was charmed to learn that you have broken with Brown. I have always thought that it was dangerous in practice to adopt any system, and that of Brown, like all the others, has sacrificed many victims. It has always appeared to me that all theories should vanish at the bedside of the sick; and woe to that practitioner who substitutes system for experience.[36]

Joseph was able to continue his work in Vilnius for another five years before war again disrupted his life and practice. Napoleon began his Russian campaign in 1812. For the Poles and Lithuanians, who greeted Napoleon as their liberator, the war of 1812 meant a brief moment of joy followed by disappointment and vast devastation. In the space of a year, more than a million combatants passed through Lithuania, bringing with them suffering, death, and epidemic diseases. In Joseph's clinic, which served as a military hospital, the pathological specimens that were part of the anatomical pathology museum were devoured by hungry French soldiers.[37] The sick devoured one another. It is estimated that about 80,000 cadavers were buried in and around Vilnius; the decimated population of Vilnius itself was ravaged by disease. The medical institutions that Joseph worked so hard to establish were ruined.

Joseph and his family had left for Vienna a few months before Napoleon and his troops entered Vilnius, but he witnessed the aftermath of the war when he returned in the summer of 1813. This provoked him to write a discourse on the effect of the French Revolution on medicine—*De l' influence de la Révolution Françoise sur des objets relatifs à la médecine pratique* (1814). His early fascination with democratic ideals had already been "shattered" by his journey to Paris in 1803. But now the effects of the Revolution had made a more immediate, personal impression. This discourse, written in a highly polemical style, gives us an interesting glimpse of how a conservative physician working in an absolutist state viewed the effects of the French Revolution on medicine.

On the whole, Joseph presented a fairly negative evaluation of the French Revolution. The sum of evils, he felt, prevailed considerably over that of good. Most universities were ruined, the book trade was almost destroyed, many excellent

---

[35] J. Frank, *Mémoires biographiques*, III. 53. 205/168.

[36] Ibid., III. 53. 245/209. In two of his letters to Dr Alexander Marcet of London, dated 9 November 1804 and 20 May 1805, Joseph mentioned his break with Brown and the influence of the journey to Great Britain. These letters are preserved in the Manuscript Division of the National Library of Medicine, Bethesda, MD.

[37] J. Frank, *Mémoires biographiques*, IV. 64. 121.

physicians died, the correspondence between physicians of different countries was abolished, and speculative thought replaced observation and experience. He attributed the spread of atheism, materialism, and Brown's medical system to the negative influences of French thought and the revolutionary spirit. Brown's system reached the Continent at the time that the principles of the French Revolution had "inflamed" everyone, especially the youth. Everyone aspired then to novelty. Authority did not count. The "great truths" discovered by the Scottish reformer were often described by his followers with the "eloquence of Danton and Robespierre"; but Brown's system was quite similar to the democratic constitutions which "appear brilliant on paper but which fail as soon as they are tried".[38] Once the "Brownian Revolution" began, medical systems succeeded one another as constitutions did within the political realm. Few physicians remained unaffected. The apparent bitterness with which Joseph viewed the effects of the French Revolution were obviously coloured to a great degree by his disillusionment with his earlier adherence to Brown as well as by the negative impact of the Napoleonic wars on public health in Vilnius.

Joseph did admit that the Revolution produced some good. It contributed to the regeneration of medical education in Paris, the application of such sciences as physics to medicine, the establishment of experimental clinics ("designed to test new remedies and new methods, treat rare or unknown diseases and educate particularly talented students"), the union of medicine and surgery, as well as to the improvement of surgery. Nevertheless, the revolutionary wars also produced and spread contagious fevers. Even more damaging to public health, in Joseph's opinion, than the revolutionary and military events was the economic crisis that they produced throughout Europe. The Continental System, Napoleon's plan to blockade England, made it difficult to import drugs. Consequently the price of drugs rose so much that only the rich could afford them. But Joseph was glad that the war was over and that for the first time in twenty years he could witness the opening of schools "without the noise of arms around".

In Vilnius, Joseph's old role as defender and propagator of the Brunonian doctrine was now completely reversed. His efforts to imbue the physicians of Lithuania and Poland with the new spirit of rational empiricism inevitably brought him into confrontation with the Vilnius Brunonians.[39] But eventually he prevailed.

Joseph's opposition to medical systems was not limited to Brown but extended to all theories and hypotheses that attempted to fit medicine within a single explanatory scheme, including those of Broussais and the German *Naturphilosophen*. This does not mean that he was opposed to theory in medicine, only that he felt medical theory and practice should reflect one another. Medical theory not based on bedside observation was purely speculative. Medical practice without theory was blind empiricism. This point of view had emerged as the core of rational-empirical

---

[38] J. Frank, *De l'influence de la révolution françoise* [etc.], Vilnius, 1814, p. 7.

[39] In the memoirs Joseph described two cases where he had to do battle with his chief opponent, the pathologist A. Bécu, over the Brunonian doctrine. *Mémoires biographiques,* III. 51. 109/88 and III. 53. 193/164. They are also described by S. Trzebiński, op. cit., note 3 above, pp. 121–2.

medicine. The many medical institutions which Joseph founded in Vilnius on this basis were to be a bulwark against speculative medicine.[40]

Joseph Frank's encounter with the medical system of John Brown illustrates well the ways in which medical theory and practice interacted, and especially those factors which influenced many young physicians in Germany and Italy to adopt that system. By organizing all of medicine around a few, simple, fundamental principles and by appealing to solidism as well as the experimental philosophy of Newton and Bacon, Brown's medical system seemed to offer a viable alternative to the humoralism against which the young physicians rebelled. Yet, at the bedside, Brown's one-sided therapy of stimulation and simplistic diagnostic categories were unable to deal adequately with the complexity of disease phenomena. At first, Joseph tried to modify Brown's system so that it could be applied at the bedside, but finally "deserted it" and all medical systems. His trip to France and Great Britain, where he came into close contact with the new scientific ethos and the spirit of rational empiricism, played an important role in that transformation.

Joseph Frank's experience was not unique, but symptomatic. It reflected the greater changes occurring in medicine at that time, especially in the evolution of clinical medicine.

[40] Descriptions of some of the institutions founded by Joseph Frank in Vilnius and of his efforts to reform the medical faculty at the University can be found in R. Kondratas, 'The medical ideas and clinical practice of Joseph Frank (1771–1842)', *Acta Congressus Internationalis XXIV Historiae Artis Medicinae,* Budapest, 1976, vol, pp. 425–32, and 'Medical Reforms at the University of Vilnius in the beginning of the nineteenth century," in Gert von Pistohlkors and others, (editors), *The Universities in Dorpat/Tartu, Riga and Wilna/Vilnius 1579–1979,* Cologne, Böhlau, 1987, pp. 87–104.

Medical History, Supplement No. 8, 1988, 89–99.

BRUNONIAN PSYCHIATRY

by

ROY PORTER*

Medical men have been cast in a singularly dim light in recent histories of the formative years of psychiatry. We are told, correctly, that the medical *ancien régime* in such traditional institutions for the mad as Bethlem—a regime of routine and standardized bleedings, purges and vomits—was hidebound, rigid, and ineffectual. In the 1750s, faced with an extraordinary attack from William Battie, Dr John Monro defended his late father's reliance, as physician at Bethlem, on venesection and emetics as the best he knew. Some sixty years later, John Monro's son Thomas was in his turn defending the identical therapies, admitting their relative worthlessness, but saying that he "knew no better". This did not convince the House of Commons Committee before which he was giving evidence. That investigating body heard witness after witness chorus William Battie's maxim that insanity responded better to management than to medicine.[1] Indeed, its Report lavishly publicized and seemingly endorsed the experiment of the York Retreat, an institution founded and run by lay Quakers, not physicians. There, medicines had been tried and found wanting, and had been replaced essentially by moral therapy: kindness, example, influence, all bearing on the mind and heart.

If the lay-dominated strategy of moral therapy thus struck a blow against the doctors, the medical profession retaliated, so Scull and others have argued, by striving to capture for itself both moral therapy and the asylums in which it was practised.[2] Medical pressure upon Parliament successfully secured for medically-qualified superintendents exclusive legal control of the new public asylums, and thus effectively turned psychiatry into a medical monopoly. In reality, however, historians continue, medicine *per se* had nothing positive to contribute to the cure of the insane. The medications increasingly deployed in the Victorian asylum—bromides, croton oil and the like—had little more to recommend them than the ancient aloes and assafoetida had; and they merely paved the way for later, no less psychiatrically inappropriate, and indeed cruel psycho-surgery. Many of today's historians have very mixed feelings about the enterprise of psychiatry *per se*. But they have been almost united in dismissing the historical antecedents of psychological medicine as, essentially, classic examples of medical imperialism, which served, wittingly or not, to mask the real nature and causes of mental disturbance.[3]

*Roy Porter, PhD, Wellcome Institute for the History of Medicine, 183 Euston Road, London NW1 2BP.

[1] Cf. Roy Porter, *'Mind forg'd manacles'. Madness in England from the Restoration to the Regency*, London, Athlone Press, 1987, ch. 4 for these developments.

[2] See Andrew Scull, 'From madness to mental illness: medical men as moral entrepreneurs', *Eur. J. Sociology*, 1975, **16**: 219–61; *idem*, 'Mad-doctors and magistrates: English psychiatry's struggle for professional autonomy in the nineteenth century', *Eur. J. Sociology*, 1976, **17**: 279–305; and more generally *idem, Museums of madness*, London, Allen Lane, 1979.

[3] See Joan Busfield, *Managing madness. Changing ideas and practice*, London, Hutchinson, 1986.

Things were not, of course, so simple. Above all, medicine itself was never homogeneous; and so, *a fortiori,* there never was such a thing as a united face of psychological medicine, or of the medicine of the mind. Doctors of course tended to share, at the deepest level, a common approach to insanity, a tendency to look to organic aetiologies, and a faith in drugs as instruments of therapy. But there the unity ceased. To general medicine, Brunonianism presented a Young Turks movement, combating the entrenched orthodoxies of the age;[4] and so it should be no surprise then that in psychological medicine too, John Brown's followers set out to challenge both the standard theories expounded at Edinburgh and other schools and the standard therapies deployed by physicians at Bethlem, in such public asylums as that at Manchester, and in the private trade in lunacy.

Research in depth would be required to demonstrate just how many, and to what extent, doctors both theoretically and practically active in insanity were devotees of the Brunonian system. John Brown himself took no special interest in mental disorder,[5] though he of course had no difficulty in fitting mania and melancholia respectively into his general scheme of sthenic and asthenic disease. In Philadelphia, that errant Brunonian, Benjamin Rush, followed Brown's emphasis upon the explanatory power of the notions of over- and under-excitation, and embraced a therapeutics which, like Brown's, set great store by the virtues of opium; but Rush's claims that the aetiology of insanity lay in the blood and the vascular system, and his conviction that heroic venesection was the panacea, were essentially unique to himself.[6] A similarly partial Brunonianism can also be found in Thomas Beddoes, whose root-and-branch attack in the *Hygeia*[7] upon the nosological enterprise of carving up insanity into a complex taxonomy of classes and species precisely followed Brown's denial of the ontological theory of disease, and his faith in its essential unity and simplicity.

More wholly and authentically Brunonian was Robert Jones's *An enquiry into the nature, causes and termination of nervous fevers; together with observations tending to illustrate the method of restoring His Majesty to health and of preventing relapses of his*

---

[4] For interpretation, see Guenter Risse, 'Scottish medicine on the Continent: John Brown's medical system in Germany, 1796–1806', *Proceedings of the XXIII Congress of the History of Medicine, London, 2–9 September 1972,* London, Wellcome Institute of the History of Medicine, 1974, 682–87; *idem,* 'The quest for certainty in medicine: John Brown's system of medicine in France', *Bull. Hist. Med.,* 1971, **45:** 1–12; *idem,* 'The Brownian system of medicine: its theoretical and practical implications', *Clio Medica,* 1970, **5:** 45–51.

[5] For Brown's own writings and a biographical account see *The works of Dr John Brown, M.D. To which is prefixed a biographical account of the author, by W. C. Brown,* 3 vols., London, J. Johnson, 1804.

[6] E. T. Carlson, J. L. Wollock and Patricia S. Noel (editors), *Benjamin Rush's Lectures on the Mind* Philadelphia, American Philosophical Society, 1981; Benjamin Rush, *Medical inquiries and observations upon the diseases of the mind,* 1812, New York, Hafner Reprint, 1962. For discussions of Rush's psychiatry see E. T. Carlson and M. M. Simpson, 'Benjamin Rush on the importance of psychiatry', *Am. J. Psychiatry,* 1963, **119:** 897–98; *idem,* 'The definition of mental illness: Benjamin Rush (1745–1813)', *Am. J. Psychiatry,* 1964, **121:** 209–14; F. Wittels, 'The contribution of Benjamin Rush to psychiatry', *Bull. Hist. Med.,* 1946, **20:** 157–66; P. S. Noel and E. T. Carlson, 'The faculty psychology of Benjamin Rush', *J. Hist. Behavioral Sci.,* 1973, **9:** 369–77; M. J. Wasserman, 'Benjamin Rush on government and the harmony and derangement of the mind', *J. Hist. Ideas,* 1972, **33:** 639–42.

[7] Thomas Beddoes, *Hygeia,* 3 vols., Bristol, J. Mills, 1802–3. For Beddoes, see D. Stansfield, *Thomas Beddoes,* Dordrecht, D. Reidel, 1984.

disease, published in 1789,[8] unfortunately for Jones just before George III's recovery from his first bout of insanity. Probably with a view to rescuing the King from imputations of being out of his mind, Jones contended that the royal disease was not "insanity" at all, but a "nervous fever". They were difficult to distinguish, he admitted, but the court physicians' reports before the Parliamentary committee clearly pointed to nervous delirium. Because this fever was "asthenic", the King's current treatment—the lowering regime of blistering, purging, etc., employed above all by the Willises—was utterly mistaken. Instead George's "debilitated state of body" required tonic treatments to build him up and sustain him: "He should now indulge in animal food, and a proper quantity of wine. Music, provided it is not too loud, will be of great service." Mental and emotional stimulus would also be beneficial: above all, access to his family should form part of a general strategy aiming to "invigorate, by all possible means, the body, and to afford every consolation to the mind."

Jones had nothing but contempt for the royal doctors. Their diagnoses had been inept; worst still, their wanton use of the term "insanity" had needlessly spread pessimism, on account of its connotations of being both a hereditary condition and an incurable disease. But as a young provincial physician whose book appeared at the worst possible moment, he found no audience and seems to have made no further contribution to interpreting or indeed treating mental conditions. Indeed, he published no further books of any kind.

A more substantial figure altogether, as a champion of Brunonian psychiatry, is George Nesse Hill. Born in 1766, Hill, unlike Jones, was too young to have been a pupil of Brown in Edinburgh (he seems to have studied mainly under Dr Maddocks at the London Hospital). He passed his career as a surgeon in Chester, claiming to have had "in early life the superintendence of two houses for the reception of lunatics", though little is known about his life. His claims to fame rest entirely upon his weighty 450-page tome, *An essay on the prevention and cure of insanity*—his only book—which came out in 1814, after, he claimed, "thirty years' experience" in handling the mad.[9]

There is no indication that Hill's treatise had any major impact upon contemporary thought or practice. Indeed, he was conspicuous in not being one of those called upon to give evidence before the Commons Committee the next year; nor was his book referred to at its hearing. And unlike, say, the writings of Samuel Tuke, Joseph Mason Cox, or Thomas Mayo, there is no sign that any of his volume's recommendations for the reform of the public treatment of the mad was ever acted upon. Indeed, therein lies his interest. For as a Brunonian writing thirty-five years after Brown's death, Hill was utterly out of step with his times. And his position as an old-style medical radical, a prophet crying in the wilderness, far away from the

---

[8] See Robert Jones, *An enquiry into the nature, causes and termination of nervous fevers; together with observations tending to illustrate the method of restoring His Majesty to health and preventing relapses of his disease,* Salisbury, Robinson, 1789. For discussion see I. Macalpine and R. Hunter, *George III and the mad business,* London, Allen Lane, 1969, 99f.

[9] George Nesse Hill, *An essay on the prevention and cure of insanity, with observations on the rules for the detection of pretenders to madness,* London, Longmans *et al.,* 1814.

mainstream, enabled him to stand as a very fundamental critic of his age. His work above all shows that medical men were by no means united in an endeavour to monopolize the control of mad people for themselves within the emergent asylum system.

Hill was by no means uncritical of Brown.[10] He had read widely in the English and Continental literature of his times, and absorbed a great deal from Struve and Pinel, as well as from Cox, Erasmus Darwin, "the acute Beddoes"[11] and others. But his basic understanding of the nature of insanity was impeccably Brunonian. Health was the state when the body's excitability— that "wonderful and inexplicable property"[12] which was a defining feature of life itself—was receiving the right amount of energy from exciting powers both external and internal ("equable stimulation" was his phrase).[13] Too much or too little excitement produced sickness, sthenic or asthenic disease respectively. That kind of sthenic condition characterized by derangement and disorientation of the mind, of conduct and speech—its symptoms were ravings, delusions, non-stop chatter, and the like—was mania. That kind of asthenic distemper accompanied by mental collapse—by the narrowing of consciousness to a repetitious absorption with *idées fixes,* by vacancy, fatuity, and stupor—was melancholia. Or, put another way, mania set in when the excessively stimulated constitution erupted not merely in such physical symptoms as fever, but in mental agitation; and melancholia resulted when too little stimulus, under-excitement, produced not only such physical signs as debility, but an under-stimulated mind, manifest in such signs as idiotism or *taedium vitae,* bordering on suicide.

For Hill, characterizing madness thus was important for many reasons. For one thing, it radically and dramatically demolished the whole taxonomic fantasy-world originally created by William Cullen, who was "less clear and decided upon the subject of insanity than on any other disease",[14] and enlarged upon by Cullen's followers, among them Erasmus Darwin and—one of Hill's particular *bêtes noires*—Thomas Arnold. All such classificatory schema were hopelessly abstract, dogmatic, *a prioristic* and idealist. "The almost endless shades of difference branched out into species by learned Nosologists and Metaphysicians", grumbled Hill, "have no one beneficial tendency, being only calculated to encumber science, disguise truth, render rugged and disheartening the paths of enquiry to young minds", and so forth.[15] The differentiae of mental illness did not identify clusters of distinct diseases with distinct and constant symptoms and signs; or rather they did so only in the crazy systems of obsessive theorists. Madness was a state, rather than an ontological entity. Insanity was a manifestation which, Hill stressed, had to be understood "symptomatically": "insanity is always a symptomatic disease".[16] It was, as it were, a barometric reading on a particular individual, depending on quite individual propensities, balances, and

---

[10] For example, he criticized Brown's views on the use of evacuants in the case of asthenic diseases. Ibid., p. 340.

[11] Ibid., p. ix.

[12] Ibid., p. 20.

[13] Ibid., p. ii.

[14] Ibid., p. 211.

[15] Ibid., p. 57.

[16] Ibid., p. xi.

responses. An action or habit—for example, consumption of heavy quantities of alcohol—precipitating manic insanity in one person would be quite conducive to the health of another (indeed, for such a toper, leaving off heavy drinking might itself trigger incurable torpor). Thus it was a nonsense to approach any understanding of insanity by proceeding as Arnold and Darwin had, by cooking up a natural history of diseases. Insanity was rather to be understood as "one species" only, as a process characterized by physiological actions and reactions, stimuli and responses.[17]

Indeed, in order to handle particular manifestations of madness, it was of cardinal importance to know the individual. Detailed case histories, conducted in depth, were essential. For insanity was not an absolute but a relative matter; it registered a discrepancy between the healthy requirement for excitation of a particular constitution, and the quantum of stimulus being received or generated. For that reason, it was vital to understand the precise concatenation of pre-existing circumstances finally issuing in mental disorder. Of vast importance was the individual's constitutional diathesis, or, in other words, his general predisposition and habit. How much food, exercise, work, mental activity was he capable of and accustomed to? Age, gender, size, habit, early diseases, education, strength, occupation, physique, physiognomy (in the literal sense, for Hill admired Lavater): all these factors and many more (Hill termed them "predisponent causes")[18] together amounted to an individual's diathesis towards mental illness. This applied in both an overall sense (how likely was such a person to succumb?), and more particularly (how would certain triggers—a brain injury, a personal calamity—affect particular individuals?). Without a detailed predispositional history, the symptoms of mental illness could be drastically, and even fatally, misread. Someone deeply agitated might mistakenly be diagnosed as suffering from mania, be given such drastic depletive treatments as heroic blood-lettings as a consequence, and thus might well become fatuous and be rendered incapacitated for life. By contrast, the expert diagnostician, with a knowledge of the diathesis in such a case, might well recognize the basically asthenic constitution and so pinpoint the therapeutic need, not for sedation and depletion, but rather for measured, exact, precise stimulus, especially to reactivate the stomach and bowels.

Indeed Hill believed, very much in the spirit of Brown himself, that it was asthenic conditions (often misjudged by superficial practitioners as sthenic) which actually posed the worst problems. Put another way, Hill, like Brown, distrusted the ready and easy recourse to depletive medicines and measures, not least the blood-letting which all too often was mistaken as a panacea in cases of frenzy and agitation. For Hill, proper knowledge of predisposing factors and the proximate causes of insanity would produce diagnoses which, in the overwhelming majority of cases would indicate that appropriately gradated and diversified stimulus which would induce that strengthening of the system which the restoration of mental health demanded.

A pillar of Hill's system, then, was the need to treat individual cases individually. Disease-centred approaches must give way to person-focused ones. Such mass and

[17] Ibid., p. xiii.
[18] Ibid., p. v.

routine treatments characteristic of the madhouse as the group annual Spring blood-let and vomit at Bethlem, defended by the Monros and by John Haslam, all of whom served as Hill's whipping boys, were quite criminal.[19]

Above all, close attention to individual diathesis would prove fruitful in prevention. Hill called his book an *Essay on the prevention and cure of insanity,* and the attention he paid to *prevention* is quite unusual in the contemporary insanity literature, with its standard emphasis on the handling of the mad once they had already been delivered to the asylum. For Hill, an ounce of prevention was worth far more than a pound of cure, and with his emphasis upon diathesis, upon organic habit, upon the need for regular stimulus as the *sine qua non* of health, he believed that it was possible to follow "precautions"[20] and regimens which set a straight course for mental health. Moreover, friends and relatives should be able to spot the tell-tale signs of insanity when they first appeared—bodily changes, alterations in the eye and countenance, shifts in manners and habits—and to intervene in time to forestall disaster. Those on the brink of mania could be soothed by changes of habitat, scene and occupation; those sliding into melancholy could be stimulated by travel, by new hobbies, by a richer diet, by enlarging their circle of friends, and so forth.[21]

No less important to Hill, another shaft of light shed by Brunonianism onto insanity, was the theory's fundamental organicist holism. Sthenic and asthenic disease, mania and melancholy alike, were attributes of the entire organic system, a single, unitary "human machine", in which the body, "together with the mind [formed] one homogeneous mass".[22] They were not just sited in, or excited by, the nerves, the liver, the heart, the blood (at this point, Hill certainly parted company with Rush), the guts or the uterus (Hill in fact says quite remarkably little about special diseases of women). They were not even principally lesions of the brain. Above all, they were emphatically not sited in some immaterial principle, some disembodied consciousness, some free-floating *cogito*.

Although Hill had the greatest respect for the insights of the associationist philosophy of mental mechanisms developed by Locke and enlarged by Hartley, he deplored metaphysical accounts of mental illness as absurd mystifications. It was arbitrary to separate mind from body, and it baffled understanding. Moreover, experience itself showed that immaterialism was just a tissue of "metaphysical cobwebs".[23] The derangement of the mind could always be shown, by the observant physician, to be accompanied by such visible organic changes as a different skin colour, squinting eyes, a racing pulse, tics, and even, Hill claimed, a quite unmistakable fetid smell absolutely unique to the insane. But these manifestations did more than "accompany": they caused as well. For Hill repeatedly argued that such bodily defects as liver complaints, irritation or inflammation of the bowels, intestinal worms and fever brought about the characteristic mental over-excitation of mania, such as the inability to concentrate on any one subject for more than a moment, or of melancholy,

[19] Ibid., p. iii.
[20] Ibid., p. 240; see also p. 236f.
[21] Ibid., p. 264.
[22] Ibid., p. 17.
[23] Ibid., p. 35.

such as anxiety, anguish, hypochondria. Because "organic functions precede mental operations",[24] because "mind itself is the product of bodily sensation",[25] because consciousness stemmed from organized existence, because thought arose from the excitation of the senses connected to the nerves, there could be no mental disease without physical diathesis, without organic disease. Hill was insistent on this point. Insanity, he argued, "is never a purely mental disease"; it "always has corporeal disease for its foundation".[26]

Characteristically, Hill favoured therapies initially and fundamentally involving the cleansing and rectification of the body: the use of emetics, laxatives and so forth. His strategy however was not routinely to deplete, but to rid the body of obstructions and toxic material. For all body waste typically produced pain, irritation and liverishness. Hill's goal was to tone up the stomach and the bowels, and to restimulate healthy body action.

Hill anticipated stigmatization as an evangel for a "cold and comfortless system of materialism".[27] He was, after all, publishing before the end of the Napoleonic War, in the aftermath of the "alarm" against the revolutionary materialist ideologies of the French Revolution. He emphasized, however, how his doctrine deserved to be embraced by all who had at heart the understanding of insanity, and the health of lunatics. For by stressing the corporality of insanity on the one hand, he removed madness from the realms of mystery, and rendered it as intelligible as all other diseases. On the other, he rendered insanity as amenable to medical therapeutics as other comparable diseases such as fevers. This paved the way for the second original feature of Hill's system: its distinctive, and highly impressive, therapeutical thoroughness. One of the noteworthy features of so many writings on insanity, in the half century preceding Hill, is how little they say about the medical management of the mad. Authors like Samuel Tuke ventured little because they thought that little was to be said. Others, like Thomas Arnold, were more interested in nosology, taxonomy and diagnosis. Still others, like Thomas Bakewell, were sitting on family nostrums which they chose to conceal (Hill found this practice quite scandalous). William Perfect would be an instance of those who used such stock items as aloes, bark and paregoric essentially as a "liquid cosh", to render the patient tractable. All of this neglect and imprecision Hill denounced, attacking the "inattention the rational method of curing insanity has experienced".[28] In his view, "too little reliance has been placed upon medical agents in the cure of insanity, and too few a number of them have been employed to obtain the end in view".[29] By contrast, he devoted close on two hundred pages to the rationale and the practice of drug therapies, not omitting such details of "efficacious medicines"[30] as how best to make up such drugs as digitalis, and thus avoid the adulterations of the druggists.

[24] Ibid., p. 50.
[25] Ibid., p. 37.
[26] Ibid., p. xiii.
[27] Ibid., p. 52.
[28] Ibid., p. iv.
[29] Ibid., p. 208.
[30] Ibid., p. ii.

Hill recognized the indispensability of sedatives in handling mania, which was, after all, the disease of over-excitation; and he devoted many pages to assessing the value of camphor for this purpose (he approved), and to showing that hyoscyamus was in this respect better for melancholics than opium, his lack of enthusiasm for which distinguished him from Brown. Even so, the thrust of his pharmacy was always towards stimulus rather than depletion. If irritation caused mania, and irritation was often caused by obstructions in the guts or the bowels, the proper course of medicines—gentle purgatives, measured emetics—would aim to stimulate the regular, lively action of the digestive parts, normalize excitation, and so restore concentration. The effects could be seen. Hill argued that maniacs were habitually costive. Their vomits brought up vast quantities of mucous phlegm; purges removed hard, indurated faecal material. Both observations proved the essentially organic determination of the diseases of the mind.

To a large degree, therefore, treating the mad was a matter of the expert management of medication, requiring "practical observers" and "medical artists" rather than "speculative philosophers".[31] Daily vigilance and flexibility were crucial, individual adjustment essential. Thus with purging, he noted, "whatever laxative is adopted, it must simply act as such day by day, being augmented, diminished, or wholly suspended, conformable to the strength of the patient and his peculiar habits and present circumstances".[32] Hill believed therapeutics to be an art peculiarly neglected, partly because the physician all too often saw himself as superior to his drugs: once he prescribed, he felt his task complete. By contrast, Hill argued, the true physician would also make up, administer, and test the effects of his own medicines.

Particularly evil was the indiscriminate use, very common in large asylums, of pacifying medicines, largely as a way of ensuring tractability. Heavy sedation, low diet, cold and inactivity would combine to produce drastic under-excitement and enervation, which would convert a sthenic into an asthenic condition. Mania would turn to stupor, imbecility, and "fixed contemplation", leading to people permanently "encased in torpor". Such melancholy would prove radically incurable.[33] Controlled and supervised medication with the right stimulants would prove a far superior technique for tackling maniacal conditions which, despite first appearances, were far more promising in their prognosis than were stupor and low spirits, simply because of the maniacs' high degree of excitability.

Herein were the existing lunatic asylums appallingly deficient. Either they neglected proper medication by design, preferring the metaphysical dogmatism of moral therapy; or they performed mass medication, rather as a missionary might perform mass baptism. Nothing was worse than the "routine of hospital practice, painful coercion, starving . . . bleeding *ad libitum*"—precisely what he found Thomas Monro and John Haslam defending at Bethlem.[34] This was only one of a whole string of complaints Hill levelled against madhouses. Indeed, he comprehensively assailed them; they were, as he quoted from John Reid, "manufactories of madness", whose

---

[31] Ibid., pp. 230, 250.
[32] Ibid., p. 342.
[33] Ibid., pp. 186, 234.
[34] Ibid., p. 225.

existence largely pandered to the convenience of relatives and friends, but which were never conducive to the good of the sufferer. Radical hostility amongst medical men to the very institution of the asylum was not unknown: Andrew Harper—interestingly another surgeon—had made a comparable attack some thirty years earlier.[35] But no contemporary questioned the rationale and the efficacy of the asylum *per se,* good or bad, so comprehensively or indeed so perceptively as Hill. Since his assault upon the asylum flowed quite directly from his Brunonian principles, it is important to examine it here.

Asylums had many individual faults, and all too many of them were run by "ignorant and barbarous keepers".[36] But the very principle of the asylum was vitiated by three fundamental flaws. First, they necessarily gave general treatment—sometimes cruel, like beatings, sometimes ineffectual, like moral therapy—whereas mad people needed utterly personal treatment. Individual diet, individual medication, individually regulated doses of light, exercise, freedom, and so forth were essential for recovery. But madhouses necessarily standardized all these items, for large facilities lacked flexibility. Overall, the effect was disastrous. "It is often more difficult to repair the mischief induced by the improper treatment of madness than it would have been to cure the original disease".[37]

Second, nothing could jeopardize chances of recovery more certainly than the herding of large numbers of the mad together. For one thing, Hill strongly suspected that madness was contagious, thanks to the odour or effluvia ("inbred air")[38] which the insane emitted. For another, the mad were in constant need of the right kind of stimulus, which would enliven their spirits and concentrate their attention. How could the company of dozens of the low-spirited, torpid, and incoherent help the individual? No sooner would he begin to regain his senses, than he would find himself overwhelmed again by the inanity and fatuity of those around him. As lucid intervals supervened, it was absolutely essential that the environment of the mad person should be tailored towards normality. In the asylum, the convalescent mad person, finding himself surrounded by lunatics, was likely to relapse into chronic insanity.

Third, the asylum perpetuated in bricks and mortar what the metaphysical theory of insanity engendered in the mind. This was the notion that insanity was a special, unique, distinct disorder, a disease, which inevitably and rightfully carried shame, odium, and stigma: in short, the notion that insanity was "tainted".[39] Not least, as a consequence, insanity was believed to be hereditary. This was erroneous, Hill argued; but the belief which denied "every cheering ray" rendered it peculiarly difficult for families to handle.[40] Because madness—unlike, say, intermittent fever—was shameful, parents or friends would not act upon it until it was confirmed and advanced; in other words, until it was too late, for what the lunatic needed above all was "early institution of the effective means of cure".[41] Then they would opt for the asylum on the principle

---

[35] Andrew Harper, *A treatise on the real cause and cure of insanity,* London, Stalker and Waltes, 1789.
[36] Hill, op. cit., note 9 above, p. iv.
[37] Ibid., p. 176.
[38] Ibid., p. 362.
[39] Ibid., p. vii.
[40] Ibid., p. xii.
[41] Ibid., p. 174.

of "out of sight, out of mind"; or, perhaps, because of the stigma would reclaim a loved one from care at too early a stage. Most appallingly of all, residence in an asylum would impress upon the consciousness of the sick person himself, at least as he recovered, the recognition that he was actually "mad". Dreadful, dishonourable and degrading, asylum confinement would create in the lunatic's mind "more terror than prison".[42] And the shock and stigma entailed would almost certainly trigger a relapse quite fatal to all hopes of lasting recovery.

In the name of humanity, and for the sake of therapeutic success, sequestration must be avoided. Brunonianism spelt out the alternative. There was nothing special about insanity: it was a condition, like all other diseases, of organic excess or deficiency. The hallucinations, the warped ideas, of the mad constituted no special problem, for such thoughts and passions were "secondary", merely symptomatic.[43] Madness was as "generally curable as those violent diseases most successfully treated by medicine".[44] No special institution, no unique mad doctor, was needed. Indeed, quite the reverse:

> The result of long attention to this matter enables me to state from the fullest conviction, and without the smallest hesitation, that *not one* recent case of madness however violent ought under any pretence whatever to be consigned to a public or private receiving house.[45]

What was required, as an alternative, was an expert regime of medication and controlled access to stimulus. The ideal doctor should have a "Lavaterian eye", should be a "vigilant observer", and should possess great "versatility".[46] This role was best conducted by a local physician, even by the family doctor; certainly by someone knowledgeable about the patient's general health and habits. Such treatment should not take place within the home, for all too often it had provided the root-cause of insanity in the first place. The ideal solution would be to board an individual lunatic either with, or under the supervision of, a regular practitioner interested in the care of the mad. Thereby all associations counter-productive of early treatment would be avoided, and the intensification of personal care would dramatically improve cure rates. Madhouses were, of course, cheaper than boarding with practitioners. But this economy was entirely false because all too often, madhouses merely confirmed madness and thus rendered the patient a lifelong charge on family or parish. True economy lay in curing the maximum number possible, and that required early intervention: "direct medical remedies can never be too early introduced, or too energetically applied".[47] Caught early, "nine out of twelve, or even ten, cases of madness admit of permanent cure".[48] The only valid function of a madhouse was to house incurables.

The stages through which Hill arrived at these conclusions are not quite clear, although they flow logically and consistently from his Brunonian attachments. These commitments may well, of course, have reflected a certain self-interest. Hill's case

[42] Ibid., p. 381.
[43] Ibid., p. 258.
[44] Ibid., p. xiii.
[45] Ibid., p. 220.
[46] Ibid., pp. 261, 361, 370.
[47] Ibid., p. 205.
[48] Ibid., p. 214.

studies, appended to the end of his volume, show that he had applied the system he advocated; he claimed to have had the superintendence of two madhouses, experience which clearly disabused him of that expedient.

What is clear, however, is that he ended up penning the most dramatic rejection of the whole emergent system of care and treatment of lunatics, and the most closely argued alternative. In spite of Hill's arguments, asylums were reformed, fortified, enlarged, rationalized, liberalized, and reformed again and again. But Hill's prediction about their necessary failure proved substantially true. Only nowadays, perhaps, are we once more seriously grappling with the possibility that the distinction of psychiatry from general medicine may have proved a vast strategic mistake.

INDEX

A

Ackerknecht, Erwin, 9*n*, 75
Adamowicz, A., 78*n*
Aicher, Fritz, 55*n*, 81*n*
Aitken, John, 44*n*
alcohol, 20, 36, 46-62 *passim*, 81
Alibert, Jean-Louis-Marie, 83
Allen, John, 23*n*, 24*n*, 42*n*, 44*n*
Allgemeine Literatur Zeitung, 65
anatomy, 12, 77, pathological 13, 18, 77, 83,
 see also pathology
archives: Bethesda, National Library of Medicine,
 50*n*, 51*n*, 52*n*, 86*n*; Edinburgh: District
 Council Archives, 38*n*; National Library of
 Scotland, 26*n*, 48*n*; Royal College of
 Physicians, 32*n*, 35-6*n*, 50*n*, 53*n*; University,
 24*n*, 30*n*, 49*n*, 51*n*
 Glasgow, University Library, 24*n*; Vilnius,
 University Library, 75-88 *passim*
Argyll, Duke of, *see* Campbell, Archibald
Arnold, Thomas, 92, 93, 95
asylums, 89, 90, 92, 96-9; Bethlem, 89, 90;
 Manchester, 90; York Retreat, 89

B

Bacon, Francis 78, 88, *see also* inductive method
Bakewell, Thomas, 95
Bamberg, hospital, 57, 58, 59, 60, 63, 64, 68
Barfoot, Michael, ix; 'Brunonianism under the
 bed: an alternative to university medicine in
 Edinburgh in the 1780s', 22-45
Bass, Johann H., 46*n*
Battie, William, 89
Bécu, A., 87*n*
Beddoes, Thomas, ix, 1-6, 9-11, 14, 18, 21, 25*n*,
 26, 41, 42*n*, 90, 92
belladonna, 81
Belloni, L., 54*n*
Berthollet, Claude, 83
Bethlem Hospital, 89, 90
Black, Joseph, 30*n*, 34
blood-letting, 23, 46, 60, 71, 72, 78, 90, 93, 96
Boerhaave, Hermann 7, *see also* iatromechanism
Borsieri, G., 85
Bower, Alexander, 15*n*
Braunstein, Jean-François, 66*n*
Broussais, F. J. V., 66, 87
Brown, Elizabeth Cullen, 26*n*, 27*n*, 28*n*, 44*n*
Brown, John: disease theory, 6, 13, 16, 48, 70,
 90; early life and education, 1-3; *Elements*, 1,
 4, 6, 24, 25, 47, 63, 64, 68, 77, 78;
 Observations, 4, politics 5, 43*n*, *see also*
 Freemasonry; teaching and practice, 4-5, 7, 26,
 35, 49, *see also* disease; excitability;
 health; nosology
Brown, William Cullen, 1, 3, 4, 24*n*, 26, 28*n*,
 44*n*, 45, 79, 80*n*, 84
Bruce, John, 30, 31*n*
Brugnatelli, Luigi Valentino, 78*n*
Buchan, Earl of, *see* Erskine, Henry David
Buchan, William, 37, 43*n*
Busfield, Joan, 89*n*
Bute, Earl of, *see* Stuart, John

C

Cabanis, Pierre-Jean-Georges, 9
Cage, R. A., 38*n*
Campbell, Archibald, 3rd Duke of Argyll, 40
Campbell, James, 28*n*
camphor, 48, 62, 81
Canguilhem, Georges, 66*n*
Cantor, G. N., 44*n*
Carlson, E. T., 90*n*
Celsus, 8
Chaptal, Jean, 83
Christie, J. R. R., 7*n*, 21*n*, 27*n*
circulatory system, 12
Coleridge, Samuel Taylor, 63
Collins, Wilkie, 22, 32
Constancio, Francisco Solano, 42*n*
Corvisart, Jean, 83, 84, 86
Cox, Joseph Mason, 91, 92
Craigie, David, 3*n*
Cullen, William, ix, 3-18 *passim*, 24, 26, 30-7
 passim, 42, 47, 49-53 *passim*, 57, 77, 84, 92

D

Darwin, Erasmus, ix, 11, 25, 92, 93
Davy, Humphry, 9*n*
Descartes, René, 77
Desgenettes, René-Nicolas Dufriche, 83
diagnostics 60, 75, *see also* symptomatology
Dickinson, H. T., 32*n*, 41*n*
diet, 37, 48, 53, 54, 55, 60, 96
digitalis, 81, 95
disease: infectious, 81; local, 13, 16, 17, 36,
 37, 48, 75, 82, 94; specificity, 6, 13, 48, 76,
 92, *see also* Brown, John; excitability;
 health; nosology; symptomatology
Döllinger, Ignaz, 65
Dover, Thomas, 47
Duncan, Andrew, 8, 32*n*, 37, 41, 42*n*, 52
Dundas, Henry, 31*n*, 40, 41

E

Eble, Burkard, 67
Edinburgh, 34-5, 40, 84; 18th-c. medical theory,
 ix, 7, 10, 23; Academy of Physics, 44; Charity
 Workhouse, 38; Incorporation of Surgeons, 40;
 Philosophical Society, 4; Public Dispensary,
 41; Royal College of Physicians, 32-9 *passim*;
 Royal College of Surgeons, 45; Royal Infirmary,
 ix, 4, 32, 35, 37-41, 49-53; Royal Medical
 Society, 4, 24, 27, 40-3 *passim*; Royal Society,
 41; University, 31, 32, 35, 39-41, 44, *see
 also* archives
Edinburgh medical and physical dictionary, 25
Edinburgh Review, 44
Emerson, R. L., 28*n*, 30*n*
Emmet, Thomas Addis, 42*n*
empiricism, 6, 7
Erregbarkeitstheorie 64, 65-9, 72, *see also*
 excitability
Erskine, Henry, 41
Erskine, Henry David, 10th Earl of Buchan, 40-1
Esquirol, Jean Etienne Dominique, 83
ether, 48